Leap of Faith

Stories of Courage from the LeRoy Butler Foundation

Leap of Faith

Stories of Courage from the LeRoy Butler Foundation

With an introduction by LeRoy Butler
Edited by Renee Wahlen Tillema

Published by the LeRoy Butler Foundation, Inc.

The information, ideas, procedures and personal experiences in this book are not intended as a substitute for the medical advice of a trained health professional. Readers are urged to consult with their own personal physician regarding any medical conditions that may require diagnosis or medical attention. Consult your physician before adopting any ideas or suggestions presented in this book. The LeRoy Butler Foundation, authors, editor and publisher disclaim any liability arising directly or indirectly from experiences presented in this book.

 Published by the LeRoy Butler Foundation, Inc., PO Box 130, Galesville, WI 54630.

Visit www.leroybutlerfoundation.org

ISBN – 10: 0-9797905-0-6
ISBN – 13: 978-0-9797905-0-8
Library of Congress Control Number: 2007932507

First Edition
Cover design: Mary Beth Bockhorst
Cover photo: Julie Geiger-Schutz/say cheese photography, Fountain City, Wis.
Printed by: Documation LLC, Eau Claire, Wis.

DEDICATION

A heartfelt thank you from the
LeRoy Butler Foundation to the following:

Tom and Jeri Bye, Oshkosh, Wis.

Brad Heinkel

Craig Kersemeier (K-tech)

Jimmy Nick at American Family Insurance

Lori Severson & family

Schneider Heating & Air

Straight Shot Express

Trig Solberg & staff
Trig's Grocery Stores

WACO (Wisconsin Association of Campground Owners)

CONTENTS

Breast cancer facts from Christina Zaleski, MS, CGC, Senior Genetic Counselor, Marshfield Clinic, Wis. and Kim Fuehrer, RN, BSN, MSM, Oncology Administrative Specialist, Marshfield Clinic, Wis.

Introduction

It was January 1997. We were playing the San Francisco 49ers at Lambeau Field. It was a real bad weather game, raining hard and the field was muddy. Fortunately, we were a team that played very good in bad weather games, especially at home. So here we are playing a team that was well respected in the league. A team with so many stars; Jerry Rice and Steve Young. It definitely was a very big game for us.

At every home game I'd run out of the tunnel and high-five everybody. I always liked doing that and being personal with the fans. But, this time was different. I'm headed out the tunnel high-fiving people and I see this lady wearing a #36 jersey. She caught my eye and I said to her, "Hey, what are you doing with a pink ribbon on that beautiful 36 jersey?" She said to me, "This ribbon is for breast cancer." I replied, "Breast cancer?" She said, "Yes, it's very serious, you know?" She said that one out of every eight or nine women are diagnosed with breast cancer each year.

So here we are in this big football game with an NFC rival. I look around as everyone is warming up and I'm talking to this young lady about breast cancer. To me that was serious. I thought, this football game is big, but this is bigger. She explained to me about mammograms, x-rays and things of that nature. She told me her mother passed away from breast cancer. So many women are stricken with breast cancer and people need to pay more attention to it. So I said to her, "You know what I'm going to do? When I retire and I have time, I am going to help raise money for breast cancer through my Foundation." She got real teary-eyed, and told me that was great. Then she said, "Go, Pack, Go!"

During that whole game, everything seemed to go our way. I don't know if it was because I talked to that young lady or not. But I remember Desmond Howard just taking that game over. He put our offense in great position to win the game. And we did win 35-14. Edgar Bennett was the best bad weather running back that I ever played with. The defense played a great game. Everyone gave 110 percent to that game. Yet, I will never forget meeting that lady and seeing that pink ribbon on her jersey.

So now, I have to keep my promise. It's 2004 and I met Lori Severson. We started to talk about some of the great things about raising money for breast cancer. At the time, I was traveling with Brad Heinkle. We went to Marshfield Clinic and Health Care Ministries in Wausau, Wis. I actually visited some of the patients and talked to them. Some of the ladies said to me, "Wow, you are LeRoy Butler, or I'm already dead." I said, "No you're not dead because this is me!" They asked me why would I take time out of my busy schedule and visit breast cancer patients. I said because I care. I have four daughters, LoReal, Gabrielle, Danielle, and Sharon. I don't want to wait for the day one of them may be diagnosed with breast cancer for me to say I want to help. I want to beat it to the jump. I want to help now.

I had a conversation with my daughters about breast cancer and explained to them about the statistics. Danielle, who is six years old, interrupted me and said, "Dad, I just want you to know how cool it is that you fly around the country to help people that you don't even know. Not a lot of people do that."

As we went from patient to patient in those hospitals hearing their stories, it dawned on me that I can use who I am, my likeness, to bring as much attention to breast cancer as I can. I felt that I was starting to make a difference.

Lori Severson came to me one day with a great idea. She suggested we go to the WACO members (Wisconsin Association of Campground Owners) and ask them to work with us to raise money for women with breast cancer. Lori is the kind of person that if you give her a good idea, she'll make it a great idea. She said we could hold fund raising events at the campgrounds. I said, "You think we can pull that off?" She said, "Sure we can!" Lori's mother, Ruth, said to us, "If you want to do that, we are behind you 100 percent." Lori's whole family dedicated their time, money and everything they believe in to go on this tour (2004 – 2006) raising money for breast cancer. Lori's sisters, Mary, Bonnie, Lisa and Linda, her brother, John, and her whole family were dedicated to this promise, and I really appreciate that.

Ruth came up with a great idea to set up a website for my Foundation. Our plan was that patients could submit their medical information and apply for financial help. We developed *www.leroybutlerfoundation.org* where people can download forms, fill them out with their doctor's information and their type of cancer or other illness. The form is then sent to us, and is reviewed by our Board.

Through the process we found that some women are forced to choose between paying their mortgage and buying their medicine. We don't want anyone to have to choose between their medicine and their life. I think we are one of the very rare organizations that actually give money directly to a patient or survivor. That makes me feel good because we do things that other organizations won't do.

An idea started to grow in my head about a book. I thought if we could find some women who were willing to share their story, we could put them together in a book about women and breast cancer. If my idea worked, the money raised through the sale of the book would go directly to cancer patients and survivors. I will always remember the lady I met at Lambeau Field wearing my #36 jersey and a pink ribbon. I hope that one day she reads this book and knows that she helped inspire me to do this.

We then began looking for sponsors to write this book for us. I met a young lady by the name of Renee who is with *InSpire Magazine*. I want to thank Renee personally for stepping up to the plate. She was not worried about time or money, but stepped forward to help with this book. She is a wonderful person to work with.

So, we started gathering our ladies whose stories we hoped to share. Lori and her sisters got together and sent out invitations to some survivors and asked them to meet with us to talk about our idea for this book. We had a great response and the interviews with the women began. I remember telling these ladies that we were going to do something that had never been done. "We are going to do a book about breast cancer and you each will have your chapter and tell your story."

I remember meeting with all of the ladies that weekend. Joyce and the people at Jellystone Warrens, Wis. rolled out the red carpet for them. Each had a free room. The Green Bay Packers played the Minnesota Vikings that week and we watched the game together. Many had never seen a Packer game before. Matt Blair from the Minnesota Vikings was there and we had a great time. We had a great fund raising day. The ladies were so excited to be a part of this. They felt fortunate to be chosen because our Foundation has helped over 400 women, and to choose this group was tough.

One young lady that didn't get a chance to be with us was Val Jostead. I really wanted her to be there because she was a very energetic, fun-loving, nice person. But Val passed away. We want to make sure her spirit lives on through this book and through everything the Foundation does.

I have dedicated who I am and what I stand for to help make sure that we get a hold of this disease. We can raise money for breast cancer research every year and that is so great. Some day there will be a cure for our mothers, sisters, and daughters.

But that research is not helping women who are sick today, right now. They have to make such tough choices. Do I pay my mortgage, or do I pay for my medicine? Do I buy groceries for my family, or do I go to the doctor? No one should ever have to make that difficult choice. Our goal at the Foundation is to reach out to women in Wisconsin and around the world who need help, but are afraid to ask. There is an avenue you can take and that is the LeRoy Butler Foundation.

The LeRoy Butler Foundation has paid for eight funerals for breast cancer patients whose families did not have the means to bury them. Cost of the funerals ranged from $3,500 to $10,000. We are more than willing to help these families because we feel that if you are a breast cancer patient, we will do what we can to help you.

Something I have always asked myself is, how can I help people? I decided to help these women because it is the right thing to do. We have also reached out to help women with leukemia. We try not to forget anybody who has asked for our help.

So many have said to me why breast cancer? I told them to think about this -- I don't want to be stuck on this earth with all these guys.

There are so many people who have helped me along the way. I would like to list a few.

I met Pat Curran, President and Founder of Straight Shot Express in Neenah, Wis. Pat's sister is a breast cancer survivor. Pat told me, "Anything you do to help women with breast cancer -- I am in." Pat's company is one of those rare ones that really tries to help others. I wish to thank Pat personally for his time and generosity.

Four years ago I met Bev Van Geffen. She has helped me organize my life by working with me to set up speaking engagements and appearances. She helped me with schedules, billings and invoices for my Foundation. I had a conversation with Bev about women being embarrassed to ask for help. I remember she said you can't always worry about what people think. Do something positive and good things will come from that. Bev understands my desire to help breast cancer survivors as she has a sister who is medically disabled. Her sister lost her job and had to sell her home. So many cancer patients find themselves very ill and in similar situations with no financial resources to get them through such a difficult time.

I have a good friend Kurt Keberlein who has also kept me focused by not forgetting about men who have prostate cancer.

At one point along this journey I have chosen, I asked myself, how can I put these women on stage to tell their story? I feel very fortunate and thankful that God has given me the ability to use who I am to give these ladies the opportunity to do just that. Until we get a hold on breast cancer, I will never stop the fight.

This book is a way for our readers to meet 15 women who have fought a very personal fight. They will tell you their very personal thoughts and experiences. Things like, how did they feel when they were diagnosed with cancer? How did they feel when they had to tell their family they had cancer?

The chapters you are about to read are going to be funny. They are going to be sad. But more than that, they will be helping somebody. So, I wish you good reading.

Remember, always put fun in your life. Always keep in mind that breast cancer does not care who you are. It is not selective in who it chooses. That is why this book is so important. We encourage women to get mammograms regularly, speak out, and become leaders in the community.

I would like to thank everyone who has given even a dollar to the LeRoy Butler Foundation. I would like to thank all those people who visited us at the campgrounds during the summer of 2006. Thank you so very much.

LeRoy Butler
August 2007

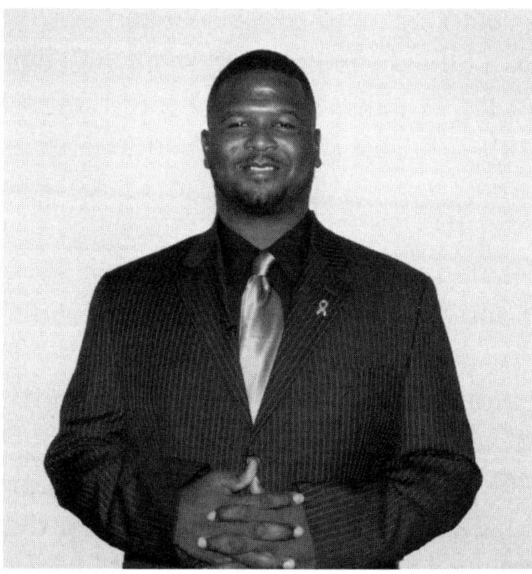

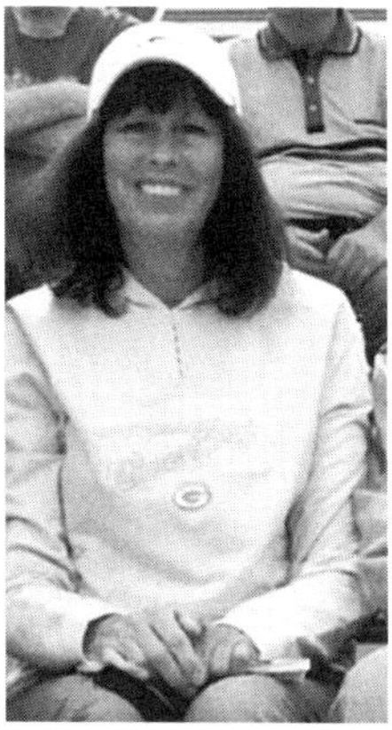

Chapter One

A Journey of Healing

By Janet Evans, Alma, Wis.

I feel honored to have been asked by LeRoy Butler to write about my experience with breast cancer. LeRoy is not someone it would be easy to say "no" to. His devotion to his family, fans, victims of breast cancer and others in need is relentless.

The moral code he lives by is steady, not giving in to the destructive behavior that is dangled in front of professional athletes and celebrities. His willingness to spend endless hours in pursuit of eliminating human suffering is an inspiration to me.

This inspiration comes not only from his present day work but also from his humble beginnings. Though extraordinarily athletic, this talent wasn't realized until later in his childhood. Much of his early life was spent in a wheelchair and leg braces. It was his determination, self-discipline, humor and positive attitude that made him a leader of the Super Bowl XXXI team.

My battle with breast cancer began two days before Christmas in 1998. Two hours after a routine mammogram, my doctor phoned me with the results and requested that I schedule a biopsy as soon as possible. In an instant my life was forever changed. Even before being officially diagnosed with breast cancer, the worst case scenarios played out in my mind. Less than a week later my fears were confirmed, although I did feel a sense of relief at the doctor's optimism. Treatment included surgery followed by radiation.

It was during those radiation treatments that I reflected on the challenges cancer dishes out. I thought about my dear friends, Ken and Sue Schumacher whose hardship had been much more difficult than mine.

Ken and Sue, along with my husband, Hale and I, spent most weekends together. We bowled, boated, played cards, partied and laughed at Ken's great sense of humor. We were devastated when we learned that not only did Sue have cancer, but that she did not have long to live.

During that time, Ken and Sue went on a cruise. When they returned, Sue described what an amazing time they had had. Her only regret was that they hadn't done it sooner. I remember thinking, "How could they have so much fun with the cancer looming over them? How could they enjoy themselves so much?" They had already learned what I would learn years later. They had faced their challenge and refused to let the cancer take their good days away from them.

A few months later they were faced with the incomprehensible news that Ken had also been diagnosed with cancer. They learned this after Ken suffered a seizure -- the cancer had already spread from his lungs to a tumor in his head. Two years was the best he could hope for. After the initial shock and numbness wore off, Ken's spirit returned. Ken and Sue laughed at themselves, cried together and cherished each other for the next two months until Sue lost her battle. What a great friend she was. I miss her dearly.

Ken began attending a support group and his optimism and humor was essential to everybody there. At one point he quit going, but returned when he learned how much he was missed and needed. It has been 16 years and Ken is now cancer free. I truly believe his positive spirit is responsible.

Remembering the dignity and grace that both Ken and Sue exhibited was something I was able to draw strength from.

Having breast cancer does not have to be devastating. It is not a death sentence and in many cases it's the beginning of life. The realization that you truly have the choice to either overcome or succumb to the cancer is yours. You can succumb by feeling sorry for yourself, wallowing in self-pity and bringing down the people around you. Or you can overcome the cancer by focusing on getting better, counting your blessings and surrounding yourself with people who can help you keep your spirits high.

Keeping positive thoughts and reinforcing a deeper gratitude for my blessings got me through that challenging time. During times of strife those optimistic feelings were at the forefront, but as things got better I slipped into a rut, taking life's pleasures for granted. Sometimes we all need a refresher course. Mine was to come two years later.

The year 2001 was not only the most difficult year of my life, in many ways it was the best.

It was after the wake of a family member when I rolled over in bed and brushed over a large, hard lump in my breast. Disbelief swept over me. I didn't need the results of a biopsy to tell me what was ahead. The following morning at the funeral, I listened as my cousin sang the Lord's Prayer, my family sang What a Friend We Have in Jesus, and watched as my sons and nephews carried the coffin. I couldn't help but wonder if the next funeral would be mine.

After returning home, a phone call to the clinic, a mammogram and an ultrasound were all accomplished that same day. The results and conversations were not the same as my previous experience with breast cancer. The optimism the doctors expressed the first time seemed to have been replaced with the cold, hard facts. I remember my daughter, Heidi, asking questions to try to get some positive feedback from the doctors. It just wasn't there and I left the clinic with an empty, helpless feeling.

Because of the size of the tumor, chemotherapy would be necessary this time, as well as surgery and radiation. A few days after the surgery, I received a phone call informing me that the final pathology report showed there was more cancer in the lymph nodes. Another surgery was scheduled.

Shock and disbelief, combined with a continual sick feeling in my stomach, seemed to consume me. I worried about the stress I was putting on my family. But mostly, I felt a determination that eventually overcame the negative thoughts. I was ready for this challenge.

Luckily, I wouldn't have to face that challenge alone. My husband's love and support has been ongoing. He has been with me through all my appointments and treatments and has been my rock, supplying me with the security that was so essential. My mother, sister and brother's unconditional love is always there.

As a mother you always want to be there for your children. The thought of not being there for them was my deepest fear. As it was, my children were there for me. My daughter, Heidi, who lived in Oregon and my son, Eric, who lived in Colorado, both moved home to help with our summer business so I wouldn't have to go through the chemotherapy alone. My son, Clint, wrote me a letter the evening after his high school graduation which I will cherish forever. Their devotion and sacrifices gave me the strength I needed.

It was the six month long chemotherapy that I dreaded the most. The nightmare stories of being so sick paled in comparison to the inevitable hair loss. I knew I would lose my hair, but I had never thought about the fact that you also lose your eyelashes and eyebrows. My daughter felt my apprehension and was determined to have a wig in place for me when the time came. When I tried on the wig that I ordered in the mail, I looked like Morticia from “The Munsters.” It definitely needed to be cut and styled. Most of the hair salons in the area wouldn't touch wigs. The few that would, wanted over a hundred dollars just for the hair cut. After countless phone calls, my daughter found an angel named Jodi Heim. Jodi not only agreed to cut the wig and style it, she refused to let me pay her. When the hair started falling out, my daughter's words were, "Just think of the opportunity you have to get to see yourself bald." This echoed in my mind and I grabbed a pair of scissors and began cutting off the rest. I remember looking in the mirror and laughing at myself. Thanks to Heidi and Jodi, it didn't seem like such a big deal.

When the doctor had described the treatment schedule six months earlier, my husband and I had circled the date of my last chemo treatment on our calendar. That date was Sept. 11. Our plans to celebrate were put on hold as we watched the planes crash into the Twin Towers and followed the events of that fateful morning as the drugs dripped through the IV. The tears of joy I had anticipated turned into tears of sorrow for the people I would never know.

The year of heartache continued when our beloved Basset Hound was diagnosed with cancer. Watching the last few months of her life ripped at our heart strings. I know everyone thinks their dog is the best, but our Alice really was the best.

With the year over, we settled back into our familiar routine. I tried to hold on to those positive feelings and to not fall back into that rut of apathy. I guess I needed one more refresher course.

It was at my six-month checkup when the doctor told me the mammogram looked the same as the previous year. An ultrasound was ordered, and the area of concern looked bad enough that I was given a choice of a needle biopsy or scheduling a complete mastectomy. They were so sure it was cancerous. For me, that was the cake taker. I couldn't comprehend what I was being told. How could I have gone through all that treatment and have the cancer reappear so quickly? I opted for the needle biopsy, which they did immediately. I left the clinic with the feeling that I had lost this battle.

That evening was surreal as a range of emotions surrounded me. There were the light-hearted moments as well. I was reminded of my son, Eric, and daughter, Heidi's, first experience with death. They were about four and five years old when they were visiting a neighbor and she told them her father had just recently passed away. Upon returning home I overheard their discussion about death. Eric was reassuring Heidi that it was alright because when you die you can go fishing whenever you want. Heidi, who wasn't as thrilled about fishing responded, "Well, when it's time to die I'm not getting in the car." Well, Heidi I'm not ready to get in the car either.

Thankfully, the following morning I received the phone call from my doctor with the results of the biopsy. The spot in question was not cancerous, but rather necrosis, which is fatty cells that have died from radiation. Elation filled me. With each step of this journey, I feel a deeper sense of commitment to God for His continual blessings.

Just a year ago I had another scare when a small, pink bump turned up on one of the incision scars which is typical of cancer. An ultrasound was ordered and once again it was determined to be necrosis. These obstacles are a constant reminder of where I've been and where I want to go.

We all have the ability to take control of our lives, to make the changes that can enrich our lives and to eliminate the negative forces around us. My brother would not allow his children to use the word "hate" as they were growing up. So many people say they hate school, hate their jobs or hate the weather to the point that they actually do. The daily tasks that we think of as drudgery now become enjoyment. The lessons I learned from my experience are not just for dealing with cancer, but rather for living a fulfilling life.

We have a campground in Wisconsin where we have been able to do some fundraising for the LeRoy Butler Foundation. It has been a joyous occasion because of the wonderful people that have been so generous with their time and money. The reluctance I sensed in the beginning by some of the campers to be involved with this event has turned into an infectious desire to do good works. It's impossible to mention all the people who make our event successful but there are a few who are always there and willing to help. My friend, Carol has worked tirelessly on this event, above and beyond what anyone could imagine. In times of need there is no one that anybody could count on more than Carol. My daughter-in-law, Nikki, has taken her talents and single-handedly raised thousands of dollars by creating baskets for our silent auction. My friend, Sue K., has been my calming influence as the event grew near. Sue A., Mary P., and Squirt all spent endless hours making jewelry and donating their efforts to the cause.

The generosity of our campers amazes me, but none so much as my friend Susie M. Her spirit of giving is second to none, so when it was her time to be on the receiving end, we all wanted to be there for her. This last fall, Susie's son was shot in a freak accident. She phoned me late that evening on her way to the hospital to inform me that her daughter was staying at the campground. She didn't want her to hear the news until she had a chance to talk to her. The desperation in her voice shook me to my core. The seriousness of the wound was critical, and the thought of Susie losing her son was unbearable. Our campers rallied around her and her family. We gave her a bracelet with the 23rd Psalm on it that one of the campers had made for our event. She wore it each day to give her strength, and as her son has recovered, she has now passed it on to another friend who is going through an unbearable time in her life. The bracelet will be passed on to others as they need it. I hope Susie never gets it back.

Many people have asked me how I found the courage to fight this ongoing battle. For me, courage is not an emotion I felt. Courage is for the men and women in the armed forces, policemen and firefighters who face death willingly in an effort to better the world. I didn't volunteer for this; I'm only trying to survive it.

I'm surprised at my emotions writing my story. Memories that have been tucked away have resurfaced as I relived my journey. More tears have fallen on these pages than tears shed over the last eight years. Surely this has been part of my healing.

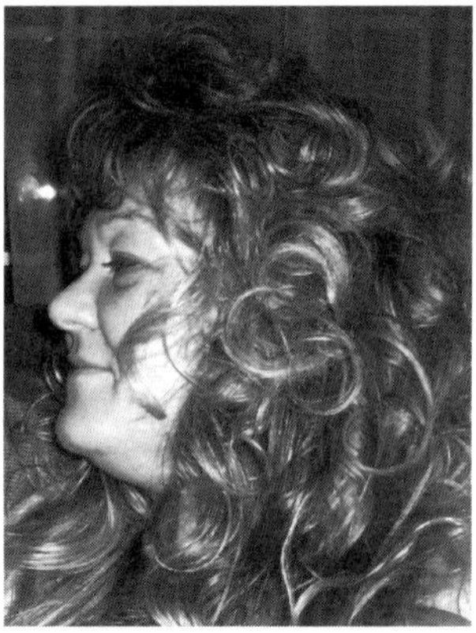

Chapter Two

The Love and Faith That Transcends Above Sickness
By Tammy Oestreich, Weston, Wis.

My name is Tammy Oestreich; I am 41 years old, married and a mother of six children from the ages of 22 to 5, two of whom are step-daughters. I own and operate my own daycare out of my home. My journey with breast cancer began last summer, in June of 2006. With school out and summer vacation about to begin, my family and I were excited for a leisurely summer break -- as leisurely as my life gets anyway. We were also anticipating an exciting summer trip for the whole family to Disney World. We were starting to make down payments on a five-bedroom, Florida vacation home. Everyone was going, including the older children. It would be my husband, myself, our six children and our new grandson.

Summer began with the usual yard work, shaping up the landscaping from the year before. This year seemed more difficult than the others had. I seemed to be more tired than usual and had more aches in my lower back and tailbone area. I brushed it off to getting older and all the extra chores in the yard. The pain got aggressively worse over the next couple of weeks. I was starting to really struggle through my daily routine of work and taking care of my family. Since my children were born I had always had an in-home, full-time daycare. Childcare is a very demanding job and I felt like I wasn't doing it as well as I always had before.

I decided to go to a local chiropractor to see if I could get some relief from my pain. There I was diagnosed with sciatic nerve pain. Over the next two weeks I did get some relief during my office visits, but the pain always resurfaced with vigor. I was abusing over-the-counter pain relievers, still with no relief in sight. One night after a treatment, in pain and frustration, I went directly to the local walk-in clinic. I was hoping to get a prescription for a stronger pain medication to take during my healing phase and continue with the chiropractor. The doctor on call was very thorough and did a complete exam including an x-ray to check for kidney stones. I left with a prescription for Hydrocodone and a new attitude that finally I would be able to get rid of this pain, get some sleep and function better during the day.

I was very wrong, not only did my pain not dissipate -- it got even worse. I received a call back from the clinic, because a radiologist saw something suspicious on my x-ray, and he wanted me in for more testing.

The weeks that followed were the most traumatic days of my entire life. It felt like I was under a death sentence. The radiologist found a dark area on my sacrum which is at the tip of the tailbone. There were lesions on my bone that needed further investigating. I was scheduled for an MRI and CT scan. I was referred to my regular family doctor. He was very concerned with my pain and the imaging that showed up on my scans. Discussing my case with a colleague, who as it is, turned out to be my gynecologist, it was recommended that I have a mammogram, because they suspected breast cancer spread to the bone.

I vividly remember the day I met with my family physician. It was like the world around me stopped and left me with this gut-wrenching pain of despair. After he talked with me about his suspicions, he asked me to phone my husband, David, and have him come down to his office. He wanted to go over everything with the two of us. The phone call was difficult. I sat there, tears streaming down my face, trying to keep my composure, telling my husband that he needed to come down and I would tell him why when he got there. Those minutes dragged by, I needed to have him take me up in his arms and tell me it was going to be OK. He was always the strong, level-headed, laid-back one of the two of us.

When David walked into the office, the doctor gave us a few minutes alone. I could hardly get the words out; I just wanted him to wake me up from this horrible nightmare. How could this be reality? After I told him what I knew so far, I could see the worried look on his face even though he did his best to hide it. The doctor came back in and went over all the further testing I would need to get a complete diagnosis. I remember my husband telling me it was going to be alright. I sat there thinking, "How could it be?" If the doctors were correct, this was the furthest thing from alright. Regardless, I knew my husband would stand at my side with me through anything. I would find out in the coming months that his job was just as demanding as mine in our fight against breast cancer.

I asked myself so many questions. Why me? How will I tell my children? How much pain will I have to go through? How long will I live and what will my children do without their mother if I don't make it? How will my husband do without me? The worst fear was the memories of losing three of my in-laws to cancer. Watching them pass away was beyond awful and knowing that this terrible disease takes so many of our loved ones lives too early. There was not any cancer on my side of our family. Why did I have to be the first?

My follow-up tests were spread out over days; the fear of not knowing for sure if I had cancer tore David and I up emotionally. I went through the regular mammogram and pap testing, along with biopsies on my breast and sacrum bone tissue. When the results were finally in, my diagnosis was metastatic HER2-positive breast cancer that had spread to my sacrum and pelvic bone through my bloodstream. I was scheduled to meet with the related doctors from the cancer center to see where we would go from here on out.

In the beginning days we told only a few close friends and family so they could be in vigilant prayer for the strength we would need to get through this. We wanted to know that every treatment and turn that we would take was covered in prayer. Looking back now, I do not know how anyone can travel this road without God's help. It is something I could not have overcome without Him. Our faith in God as a healer and deliverer is what kept us strong.

By the time I was diagnosed, 10 lesions were giving me excruciating pain; I could not walk, stand, sit or lay without pain. From a medical perspective my future looked dismal, but God had other plans.

Breast cancer is such a personal and emotional disease; it is like you feel that you are or will be less of a woman having this disease. Through God's grace, it turns out that you become a better woman going through it -- a better person, wife, mother, and friend. Still, I really did not want everyone to know about it at first. We talked with our older children, which was difficult. We didn't want to scare them with the reality of what we were facing. Then we carefully explained to our 7- and 5-year old, that Mom was sick and that I could be for awhile. It was less difficult with the help of some great coloring books at the cancer center.

The hardest thing was to tell our parents. We knew they would be devastated. After explaining that we were determined to fight back with homeopathic healing and that we also had a great group of physicians that were providing us with the newest and best treatments too, some of their worry was alleviated. I simply said that I was not going to die this way. God was going to heal me and guide me through this. My will to be here to love my husband, children, family and friends was what helped me in my war against this deadly disease.

Once the word was spread, hundreds of friends, family, churches and people that didn't even know us rallied with us and prayed for us. Their support was very important. Even though I had the best doctors that encouraged me all the time, at some point they still needed to give me the negative side, that I will have to have these treatments and they may not even help. That I will need treatment for the rest of my life and eventually, I will die from this deadly disease. *IT IS VERY HARD TO SWALLOW!* That was my reality of someone with Metastatic Breast Cancer. I knew God was bigger than any medical prognosis. I knew that God would not leave my children without a mother, but if even the littlest seed of doubt takes root within you, it can bring you crashing down. Instead it brought me to my knees in prayer. I prayed almost around the clock. I retrieved any information I could find on natural healing, from books and via the Internet. I researched the dos and don'ts of breast cancer. I would need to make a complete change of lifestyle to get a foothold on my disease.

Reluctantly and sadly, I had to give up my daycare children, and our second income, which was even more difficult. There were three children I had taken care of from birth. I also had just started with a fourth baby and was to have a fifth in late November. I ran a very loving and prosperous daycare. I enjoyed every day, even the difficult ones; it was my passion and I felt, my calling. I decided that I would have them back in my home as soon as I was well enough. The parents were all very kind and went above and beyond in keeping my positions open with their children for a later date, when I could take them back. I am sure it was difficult for them, not knowing what the future may hold.

So this is where I began my healing. First I fasted and prayed for about a week straight to cleanse my body and soul. I lived on pure bottled water, organic juice and every vitamin and supplement available to me that I had researched and that was recommended for cancer. I had to buy them as I could afford them. It was quite expensive, but my husband and I knew we needed to just do it, so we spent whatever savings we had left at our local health food store. I stopped taking my prescription painkillers because they were only poisoning my system further. I iced my pain and prayed for relief when the icing didn't work. God never let me endure more than I could handle. Amazingly, I started to feel better. My system purged some pretty nasty build-up of toxins, my body was cleansing itself and my immune system was being restored. That is when my energy level skyrocketed. Some nights I never slept, and I was not even tired the next day. My body was super-charged and on its way to healing.

Once the cleanse was over, I stuck to a very strict diet of organic fruit and raw or steamed vegetables. Slowly I added rice milk, legumes, grains, nuts, baked fish, organic chicken and eggs. No sugar, white flour, red meat, pasta, bread, dairy or junk food was allowed. The problem with eating healthy is that it is very expensive, which is a sad thing. There is something wrong with our way of life when it is cheaper to eat foods that are not very beneficial, or can even be harmful to the body.

Going from a second income of about $16 per hour, 8-10 hours per day, down to nothing, leaves a pretty large hole in your finances. My husband could not make up the difference even if he tried since he was already putting in a 10-12 hour day and getting paid a salary for it. So we had to start making some choices about what we could pay and what we had to leave unpaid. The stress of the ongoing stacks of bills not getting paid was getting higher with each passing day. Every trip to the mailbox left us more frustrated. Unless you have had a medical illness that leaves you unable to work, you can not know how difficult things can get.

The medical bills started coming in from testing, surgeries, prescriptions and this is after insurance has paid their share. It is phenomenal the cost to have cancer treatments. I did not have to have regular chemotherapy, but I had an intravenous treatment like chemo and the cost was $3,000 every three weeks. My radiation that I had to have was 10 days long, 10 minutes each time and almost $17,000. If I had not been doing my natural healing along with my medical treatments, I may have had to have several rounds of radiation. My breast cancer is hormone receptive, so I needed to have surgery to have my ovaries removed, a lumpectomy, a port put in and the costs were way beyond what we could afford, even with insurance. Our insurance year ran from Sept. 1 to Aug. 31, so once our deductible was satisfied and our out of pocket maximum met, we had to start all over with new ones. Our out of pocket total so far, is over $10,000 and it hasn't even been a full year since my diagnosis.

It was so stressful to have bills that we couldn't pay piling up. While I was trying to get better, our financial situation just continued to get worse. When talking to bill collectors when they would call, I tried to explain that there just wasn't hardly enough money to cover our regular monthly bills, let alone pay something each month to each place where we had medical bills. I didn't want to jeopardize my health by taking on too much too soon, but I just could not live like this.

I started taking my daycare children back slowly to try and get caught up. I talked it over with my husband and he didn't want me to overdo it either, but he said it had to be my decision. I know he really just wanted me to concentrate on getting well, but he knew that I have this stubborn side to me, that I would do it my way regardless. I trusted God for His healing and I would trust Him for the energy to make it through each day of work. I felt like at least this way I could help my husband and have some control over our situation, instead of going into financial ruin.

My mother phoned me one evening to talk about an article in her local paper about the LeRoy Butler Foundation and what they did. She knew how hard we had been struggling with our finances and she wanted to give me the contact information so that we could ask for help. Well, asking for help is a hard thing to do. We had always paid our bills and were brought up to be responsible adults that made our own way.

We did let some time pass before contacting the foundation, whether it was pride or just feeling like there were other women with breast cancer that needed the help more than us. I finally wrote a letter explaining our situation and waited for a reply. Not very much time had gone by when a member of their foundation contacted me. She explained that they would be issuing a check and getting it out in the mail. The same night, LeRoy Butler phoned with a follow-up call and talked with me about our situation. I remember how nervous I was when he called, how encouraging he was and how touching it was that he would take the time to make a personal phone call. He explained that he would get a check out to us immediately. He stood behind what he said because we received a check, next day air delivery, and with it we were able to get caught up on our auto loans. We should not have been surprised that in an answer to prayer, God had provided though this caring foundation, the exact amount of money that we would need to get our auto loans up to date.

The Leroy Butler Foundation gave us hope in our hopeless situation and helped us when we could not do it by ourselves. A lot of people donate money to different organizations that do research for cures, but this foundation gets the needed funds directly to the cancer patient that needs it so desperately. Giving to research is important, but if you want to directly help cancer patients, this is the place to donate.

Since then, we still have many unpaid bills but are starting to make small dents. I am back to work full-time with my daycare. I take care of two infants five days a week, 8-10 hours a day, and three toddlers part-time. We now try not to worry and give it to God in prayer. We are moved beyond words of expression by the compassion our co-workers, friends, families and relatives have shown with emotional and financial support. Now when we go to the mailbox, along with our bills, we receive cards full of encouragement and gifts of money, gift cards and a hope for our future. Some donations have even come signed anonymously -- a friend. We are very touched by everyone's generosity and thoughtfulness. God takes care of us on a daily basis and to Him and many others we are so thankful.

Even with all the help we have received financially and with going back to work, we are still behind. Our hearts and empathy go out to all the patients that haven't had help like we have. How do they make it? What about the ones that can't go back to work because they are too sick? How do they cope with the endless bills? These suffering women, fighting for their lives, only to be daily dealing with the on-going debt, when they need to be concentrating on getting well! Our heart aches for them. We lift them up in prayer and will do all we can to help The LeRoy Butler Foundation continue their efforts for a great cause.

A wise, elderly lady from my church that had her own battle with breast cancer and won, told me once and reminds me often, that the big "C" is not cancer, it is Christ. He is the covering that is needed to heal, deliver, and rise above all sickness. It's all about your relationship with Him and eternity; life here is short. I think that it's also about courage to face each new day with a good and positive attitude.

It's about a loving husband that will clean, cook, do laundry and anything to help you, even after he has put in a 10-12 hour work day. It's about great doctors that will encourage, research your best options, and give the best medical treatment, even when you can't pay the entire bill. It's about smiling, hard-working nurses that care for you and will stay on the phone for hours to get your insurance company to cover a treatment you need. It's about friends that will stop by with an uplifting visit and end up helping you clean your house or hold a baby for you. It's about a mother that has driven two hours, putting her own life aside, to come to your house and do anything you need her help with. It's about a mother-in-law that has traveled a similar road and would drop everything to watch your children. It's about a foundation like LeRoy Butler's that will get needed funds to cancer patients that desperately need their help. It's about all the people that have given to us so generously, even when they don't have a lot to give. It's about moms of your daycare children that will make meals and desserts for your family and give your tired husband a break. It's about how they rally around you, encourage, and wait for you to get well, and kindly find alternative care when you have appointments and are sick. It's about the babies I take care of, even though some days are a lot of work, when they smile and coo at you, it brings tears to your eyes. You fight harder so you can be a part of their special little lives. It's about toddlers you take care of that trust you and make you laugh, and making them giggle and laugh when you play with them. When they are excited to come back, you know you are making a difference. It's about my own children that love me and need me for so many reasons, but especially to hug and kiss them every morning and night. To all these loving souls we say thank you from the bottom of our hearts!

Every breast cancer survivor has many battle wounds, physically and emotionally, but that is what builds you courage, makes you stronger, and gives you the strength to carry on. Your life is more precious because you realize that every day you have is a gift from God, a bonus round in life. Don't ever give up; every day is a new day! God will help you and bring those to you to help when you can't do it yourself. Draw closer to God, love your husband, children and everyone you know with all you have.

Appreciate those that stood by you through the emotional mood swings, tests, treatments, radiation and surgeries, because some days it couldn't have been easy for them. When I was diagnosed I asked, "Why me?" I know now it was for many reasons, maybe so I could tell this story -- and I will with zeal and devotion to help anyone I can. Thank you to all who have helped me and continue to help me fight with courage, strength and hope.

Cancer care is both a science and an art. It is important to develop a dialogue with your cancer care providers and take an active role in determining which treatment is best for you. Advocate for yourself by becoming your own expert and researcher of information. Healthcare providers who really listen to their patients learn as much or more from their patients as patients learn from their healthcare providers. Together, you help remodel care for the future through the wisdom gained and sharing of experiences.

- Kim Fuehrer, RN, BSN, MSM, Oncology Administrative Specialist, Marshfield Clinic, Wis.

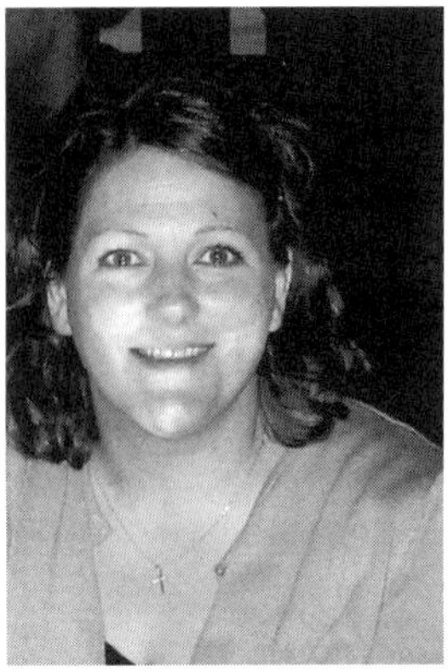

Chapter Three

My Journey Through Cancer
By Stefka Meddaugh, Granton, Wis.

Where do I start? I went in for a mammogram on May 10, 2005. They did the regular one year check-up and spotted an area that wasn't clear. So they did an ultrasound and then a biopsy on my left breast. This turned out to be a benign breast disease that they call Fibroadenoma non-cancer lump. Within a few days they called and said everything was fine. I was still sore from the biopsy and had broken out in redness – which they think may have been a reaction from the ultrasound-guided biopsy. This was still sore even a few months later.

Yet, something didn't feel right. I went to my primary doctor to see what was going on. There was a lump that would come and go, and it seemed to be quite large. The doctor told me maybe it was my hormones working and making my breast sore because everything on the mammogram turned out to be OK.

By November of 2005 I started noticing that I wasn't feeling well and I had lots of breast pain. But, I just chalked it up to holiday stress, with everything spent and everything due after the holidays. And anyone I talked to about this told me, "Don't worry, it couldn't be cancer, because cancer doesn't hurt."

Well, after the holiday I had spasms and this weird burning sensation in my breast. It was also tender to touch. I just couldn't take the pain anymore. That was it. I called the radiology department and was persistent that I would like another mammogram done. So they set me up for a mammogram, noticing that I just had one about six months ago. I explained to them what was happening. Due to a family history of breast cancer, I was scared. I was determined to get in. I wanted a mammogram and an answer – this time I took my husband along.

So on Jan. 27, 2006, they set me up for a mammogram, which showed an abnormality. They set up another appointment on Jan. 30 for a mammogram ultrasound exam, but it did not show the full extent of the mass because of the density of the breast. So again I was set up for an MRI on Feb. 9. The MRI showed the mass to be larger than what they saw on the ultrasound. So they did an ultrasound-guided core biopsy and drained multiple cysts.

I remember lying on the table in this small room. A few more doctors came in – I felt scared and kept trying to understand what was going on, but did not really understand the medical terms they were using. I felt the pressure from the biopsy. I was lying very still, just wishing that my husband could be there to hold my hand, but instead the tears kept running down my cheeks and into my ears. I felt like I was in a daze -- counting the dots on the ceiling -- until they were done. They didn't say much, so I thought I was overreacting and they were just being cautious.

I went home and a few days later my world seemed like it was going to end. Who would know just one phone call could change everything!

Feb. 14, 2006 – Valentine's Day

How my life changed when I was diagnosed with breast cancer. I remember my primary doctor calling me the morning of Feb. 14. The tone of her voice was different. My doctor asked me, "Do you have someone there with you?" Those words just broke my heart. I knew something was wrong. She told me she had some bad news. My heart seemed like it had stopped. She told me she needed me to come in because the test came back and it tested positive for breast cancer. They would like to get treatment started. I hung up the phone and just sat there. Of course, the first question was, "Why? Why me?"

The only thing I knew about cancer is that it is a killer. I'd lost my father and mother both to cancer, among others. I saw the pain they went through. I was terrified of what was going to happen to me. My heart started racing. I called my husband at work and told him that the clinic called and they wanted me to come in, that it was breast cancer. I heard silence, and then crying. "I will be right there," he said. It seemed in a flash he was there by my side.

We went to see the clinic consultation, the surgeon and oncology department. They set me up with a bone scan, heart scan and blood work. They told me I had cancer in the left breast and that it was quite large. We talked to the surgeon and I gave him a little history of family members with breast cancer and ovarian cancer. He was concerned and thought it would be best to meet with a genetic counselor. It was very important for the decision of my surgery. If positive as a carrier, we would be looking at a mastectomy with both breasts and removal of the ovaries at some point. The cancer would have a higher risk of coming back.

Then we talked to the oncology doctor, and he recommended shrinking the large tumor first. So he suggested the neoadjuvant chemotherapy. The treatment would be administered every three weeks for six cycles, then surgery, followed by radiation for the completion of the treatment.

My husband and I were so overwhelmed. At that time I don't even think I heard exactly what they were saying. Everything seemed to be going so fast. My anxiety was so high. I heard cancer and all I thought about was, "Am I going to die? I'm not done here, my family needs me." My husband didn't know what to do for me. So I asked him if he would take me to see the priest. It was like you turn to God when something seems to go wrong. My life seemed to flash before me. I started writing letters to my family, my husband and our children, just to say how much I loved them.

Feb. 20, 2006 – First Treatment

I was scheduled early in the morning to get a port placed in to make the treatment easier. I remember driving there begging and crying that I couldn't do this. I decided not to have the port put in because I felt like I couldn't think for myself. With my anxiety being high, and crying a lot, I was physically and emotionally tired. What made it even worse, I didn't want to eat or drink anything. I felt like I was a burden to my family. I don't know how I even cried. Thinking that I couldn't make it to tomorrow, all I needed was just a few more hours of sleep to be closer to the next day. It was like I didn't even know who I was. I watched as they put poison into my vein to help me. Then I remembered something that stuck in my head when I was talking to a priest in the hospital. I kept asking him to help me understand. He told me, "Stop trying to find God and let Him come to you." And that is what I seemed to do.

About 14 days into my first treatment I started losing my hair. I knew something was happening when my head started to itch a lot.

There were times no one could hear me or see me crying. I would stand in the shower until the water ran cold so I didn't have to have anyone watch me be sad. I was scared when my hair started falling out and I would watch it go down the drain. No one knew the anger and pain I felt. I then found it difficult to look at myself in the mirror. So I asked my kids if they could shave my head. My daughter just cried. I tried not to cry when my son, Matthew, shaved my head, with a little humor. Little at a time and shorter until it was gone. I cried and laughed. I noticed that I didn't have a perfectly round head.

March 14, 2006 – Second Treatment

I wasn't as scared because I had made it to the second treatment and knew what they were going to do and kind of how I would feel. But when I checked in the tears started running down my cheeks. Here I was, only to start all over again -- being sick for two weeks and one good week -- to start again.

I had a hard time keeping food down. Nothing smelled or tasted good due to the chemotherapy, which kills some good cells. At this time I was feeling bad for myself. I had my sister tell me that there is always someone in worse pain than me at this moment. This is true. But it wasn't that I was trying to be selfish, my concerns were for my family. Did I teach them what they needed in life? There were no guarantees that the tumor would shrink and the chemo would work. I was mad that I was a woman.

It wasn't just me that was bothered by the cancer. I watched my daughter, my sons and my husband crying for me. Worrying about their jobs and wanting to be there for me. Wondering why this was happening to me. I wanted to be strong, but I just couldn't at first. You go through being angry and blaming everything. Lots of times I couldn't understand things because maybe I didn't want to. Only if someone had good things to say – I just wanted to hear positive things. Even from the doctors.

April 3, 2006 – Third Treatment

I agreed to have blood drawn for the genetic test. I was scared to know the results of the test, not just for me, but for my family and concern for life and health insurance. I had to wait four weeks for the results. It was starting to get hard to have my blood drawn because my body was getting weak from the chemo. My hands were sore and bruised from them trying to find a spot to draw the blood. My white blood counts started dropping low, which made me at higher risk for infection following the chemo treatment. The next day I would come for a shot to reduce the risk of infection and help the counts go up faster so I could keep my treatment on time.

The shot made me have lots of aches and bone pain the next day. I couldn't even get up or turn my body; I was in pain. It seemed things were getting worse. Because of my counts being low, I couldn't take a chance of anyone coming or going anywhere and had to wear a mask to protect myself from germs.

Waking up early crying to myself, I realized all the simple things in life seemed to make me happy. Like sitting by the patio window watching the sunrise, taking a walk and feeling the warm sun. My daughter had a camera on the table. The sunrise looked so pretty, the sun peeking through the clouds. So I took a picture of the cloud, it looked like a cross. The clearer it got, it looked like an angel setting free a dove! I thought of that as a sign to me. I was hurting and God had sent an angel.

April 26, 2006 – Fourth Treatment

I went in to see the surgeon; he said the mass is decreasing in size, so they wanted to put in an ultrasound-guided clip placement – in case it shrunk completely. But my treatment had to be delayed a week because I had bronchitis. I never thought I could have made it to my fourth treatment. The more the chemo increased, the more it made me tired and nauseous and it became painful. I had problems keeping food down; it seemed one thing led to another. I tried hard not to be sad. I eventually lost every single hair on my body, including my eyebrows and even my eyelashes.

My husband has helped so much, from listening to me cry and me telling him my fears. He was there at every doctor's appointment to comfort me. He would tell me, "Tough times can't last forever." I kept saying, "I'm OK." But he knew I was hurting. So my family, knowing I love being outdoors, they started a vegetable and flower garden for me. But I had to be careful; I had two more treatments to go.

May 24, 2006 – Fifth Treatment

I finally got my results from the genetic testing. It came back "negative." This helped me make a decision. So everything was going as planned. I started getting swelling in the left side of my body and some numbing. Some was partly from the medicine and they also found kidney stones and a few cysts causing the pain.

June 21, 2006 – Sixth Treatment

Thank Goodness I made it this far. Before my treatments would start I would go to church early, just to light a candle and to sit in silence and pray. I would say, "Just give me the strength and the rest is in your hands." It seemed to comfort me through my treatments. I had many challenges from my chemotherapy, from being sick and loss of appetite, to low counts. We went and talked to the surgeon and I told him about my fear of being put to sleep. We also talked about the genetic test that came back negative. We then scheduled surgery in July.

July 11, 2006 – Day of Surgery

My family all got up early to go with me. Driving to the hospital, everyone was silent. No one knew what to say. I checked in and in a few minutes they called my name. I kissed my family and didn't want to let go. I said, "I love you." I was taken to a room to change and get the IV started. The anesthesiologist came and started talking to ease my fear. Then I remember them wheeling me into the operating room. It seemed like a few minutes and I was waking up. I was so thankful to see my husband standing there. The surgeon came in and said they did a segmental mastectomy, had removed nine lymph nodes and placed in a drainage tube. He said everything went well. The nurse told me that my family was waiting to see me.

Aug. 1, 2006 – Drainage Tube Removed

Having the drainage tube so close to your nerves was more painful than I thought. Every movement would make me cry. I couldn't sleep either, it would hurt so much to toss and turn. So I had to be extra still and lie there so the tube wouldn't slide out. The tube was only holding by a thread and tape. Time didn't seem fast enough until they did finally remove the tube.

Aug. 21, 2006 – Radiation

I went everyday for 33 treatments of radiation, with one week of additional boost. Radiation didn't seem as bad as chemo. I was in and out in about 10 minutes at the most. But I did have some side effects, such as skin changes -- it felt like sunburn. And I had some loss of appetite and tiredness. I think a lot came from driving back and forth. Thank goodness for my sons, Adam and Matthew, for driving me everyday. The plus side of the radiation was that my hair was starting to grow back!

Oct. 29, 2006 – Last Day of Treatments

I am a survivor – I'm alive!

Thank you to my daughter, Deanna, for making me a chocolate cake to celebrate the end of my treatments.

I kind of look back now – they say if you've ever done something you were afraid to do, you have courage. I guess I really know that now. And my strength seemed to come from the family support that kept me going. They gave up a lot for me. I am grateful that they were there and helped each other when it came to being a family. Knowing that they were all there for me – supporting me – I know helped me to get through all the treatments and all the hard times when I wanted to give up. I was told many times that I was lucky to have boys that were so caring and helpful. Thank you to them for all they did. And thank you to my daughter for understanding what my body meant to me. Thank you to my husband for being my rock -- you were my strength.

The rest of my family, you all helped the time go fast. You were my support. I'll never be able to thank all of you enough. You took up what I couldn't do.

My family told me that I had given them so much that it was time to care for me.

Even the smallest kindness can help. But sometimes it wasn't like that; people would sometimes try and avoid running into me. I was always scared when they said things were going to feel different. I thought they meant the chemo – not the people. But it happens all around – in public, at home and with me. It's like I know what they were thinking – what do you say to someone who is sick?

It was hard for my sister to tell me what to expect from her breast cancer because she had "chemo-brain." She would forget things and didn't remember much after her treatments. This really does start to happen. She is a survivor of four years now and counting.

I was so thankful when I took a walk and could feel the breeze in my hair -- I cried, but this time it was a happy cry. As for now, there are times when I'm still recovering and feel pain and wonder how to cope with the changes to my body.

I know I have changed and came out stronger. And I also know differently that cancer doesn't mean death.

This is my story.

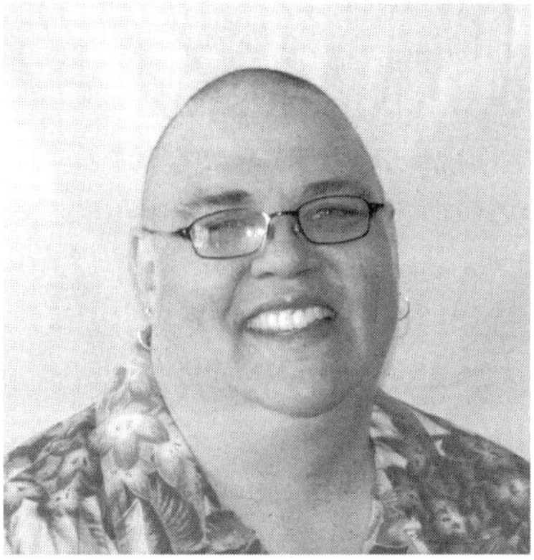

Chapter Four

A Reason to Hope

By Kimberly Lindau, Wautoma, Wis.

Dear Leroy,

On March 18 of 2005 I was diagnosed with stage 3 of stage 3 breast cancer. I had a radical double mastectomy on March 23. I have gone through 3 surgeries and numerous tests since then, and will have to keep going through this until at least 2010. As you can imagine my doctor's bills are huge. I am writing to you after reading an article in the Waushara Argus about your foundation. Because my cancer had advanced to such a late stage every precaution is being taken to hopefully prevent the cancer from returning. As a result of everything that has been going on I am only able to work 24 hours per week, and I have so many doctors bills and gas expenses I am drowning, not to mention mortgage payments, car payments and all of the normal things that go along with life. I am not very good about asking for help and have quite literally tried to receive help from so many organizations. The American Cancer Society sent me two gas cards for $20.00 a piece, which helped get me to about 6 of my 48 radiation treatments. My friends and coworkers at the hospital have donated well over 300 hours of PTO time to help me offset the time off that I have had to take. The drugs I have to take are mounting up quite an expense. At one point I was willing to give up because I know I am a burden to those around me, especially financially. After a lot of research done by friends and family it is sad to say that there really aren't many organizations that actually help people survive this life altering experience financially. Most of the funding is spent on research, which I obviously am grateful for, as my life has been extended for at least a year and 6 months

as result of all the research. I guess that I am looking for help from every organization I or my family and friends come across, and yours is the only one we haven't tried...We didn't know that your foundation was out there, so I am giving it a go with the hopes of any help at all...even if it can only be a gas card.
I have no problem sending you copies of my diagnosis, bills or whatever you need to know that I am truly being honest.
Thank you for your attention,
Kym Lindau

(A copy of Kym's e-mail sent to the LeRoy Butler Foundation in September of 2006.)

It all began with a phone call on a Friday night to one of my friends in Southern California, Sue Newton. She said that she had breast cancer and was going in for a lumpectomy! Needless to say, I was shocked. Sue is a 10-time All American softball player and was big in the world of fast-pitch softball for a number of years. I'm not sure why, but it caught me by surprise. I told her that I had a lump, but was kind of blowing it off because there was no history of breast cancer on either side of my family. My mom and sister had lumps removed, but they always turned out to be nothing.

On Monday I called and scheduled a mammogram for the following Thursday, March 17, 2005. Something popped up on the test and an appointment was made to see a surgeon on Friday, March 18. I worked in the emergency department at a hospital and I was very familiar with the surgeon, so I was comfortable with him. He took a biopsy and I carried it back to work in a brown paper bag for the pathologist to look at. He explained to me that if it was in fact cancer that I would have to decide on what to do because there was also a suspicious spot on my right breast, but it was too small to actually biopsy. I was pretty calm as I left the surgeons office.

Once I was in my truck I called my mom who was at church at a meeting. I told the secretary that it was an emergency and to have my mom call right away. As soon as she called back, I became hysterical and so did my mom. I know that she was trying to hold it together, but she had already buried one child, my only brother, Mark, who was killed by a drunk driver. I'm sure that a million things were running through her head at that time, too. At that point, all I could think about was that if it was cancer, at least it was me instead of my younger sister, Sue, who has a son, Cody, and a husband, Tom.

I told my mom what the doctor had said and that I was on my way in to work with my biopsy in a brown paper bag. Within the hour, my surgeon called back to tell me that it was in fact cancer. My bosses took me into their office to get the news from the doctor. We all just kind of sat there and cried. I didn't really know how to react because everything was coming at me so quickly. My doctor told me that he would see me on the following Wednesday, March 23 for surgery. He told me to think about whether or not I wanted both breasts removed and I told him it was a "no-brainer." Take them both!

The rest of the day seemed so surreal. I was truly walking around in a zombie-like state. My roommate, Tammy Gee, who also works in the ER, was in the office when I got the news and she and my bosses did a good job of calming me down. As soon as I recomposed myself I went back to work. My co-workers knew that something was happening and I gave them the news. It was all so overwhelming! In five days I was going in for double, radical mastectomies! I had never even imagined that something like this could happen to me! I was an athlete, my parents had already experienced burying a child, and now they could possibly have to do it again.

Those four days leading up to my surgery were some of the longest in my entire life! I had named my tumor "Emily," I'm not sure where that came from, but we all joked about it during those four days. I would sing songs like, "Ding, dong, the tumor is dead; Emily's gonna lose her head." I know this sounds morbid and bizarre but it was definitely my coping mechanisms taking over. I told people to be careful what you wish for because you just might get it and it might not be the way you want. I had always wanted a breast reduction and wanted to know what it would be like to shave my head, well I guess now I was getting the things I had "wished for!"

The day finally arrived. My family and my roommate were there at my side from the moment I arrived at the hospital. We all prayed together, which was only appropriate because my dad is a Lutheran pastor, and we knew that people were praying for me literally all over the world. My mom told me on the way to the surgical center, "They are going to have to tie you down because of all the people who are holding you up to God right now!" I was scared to death, but I knew that God had a plan.

While I was being prepped for the surgery, I asked the surgical team if they would weigh my boobs, they all laughed, but knew it was me, and they realized I was serious. After all, I had been carrying them around with me all of my life and was rather attached to them! I wanted to know what was going to happen to them. We were all laughing at that point, which was good. I told them that I had named the tumor Emily, and that they were going to "take care of her" for me.

When I woke up in the recovery room it finally hit me what I had just been through. It dawned on me that I actually could have died. I realized that potentially I could still die. I hadn't thought about dying; actually I hadn't thought about it since the day I called my mom to tell her what was happening. My attitude was, "It is what it is," nothing more, nothing less. I have a bachelor's degree in psychology and know that attitude has a lot to do with recovery. I know that mind, body and soul are so intertwined that if one doesn't focus on the whole, the whole doesn't always get better.

After being brought up to my room, my surgeon came in to see me. The first thing I asked him was, "Am I going to croak?" To which he replied, "No." I then asked him, "Did it metastasize?" And again he said, "No." He then went on to explain that I had the faster growing of the two types of breast cancer and that I was very lucky. The tumor that we all thought was 2.5 centimeters was in fact 8 centimeters, which is quite large, about the size of a tangerine. He also explained that they had removed 12 lymph nodes. Nine from the left side, and all were cancerous and the size of golf balls, and three from the right side that had no signs of cancer.

My doctor went on to say that he had cut out all of the "big stuff" and then the chemotherapy and radiation would take care of all the microscopic stuff. He also explained that the cancer had gone to stage three of stage three and that for at least the next five years they would have to keep a very close watch on me because of the possibility of a reoccurrence. I would have to be checked out about every three months.

I had four drain plugs that I had to empty every day, several times a day. I had to record the amount each time. The pain from those four plugs was excruciating. My doctor said that I would probably have them in for a week or two. I thought, "No way!" I had the first two removed about five days after surgery and the last two about four days afterwards. It was proof positive that my attitude was helping. Every time I felt the pain I would tell myself that I was getting better, and I firmly believe that's why I didn't have the drain plugs for the period of time that I thought I was going to have them.

The weekend before my first chemotherapy treatment I had my sister, nephew and brother-in-law shave my head. I thought it would be less traumatizing than to wake-up with clumps of my long hair on my pillow, or in the shower drain. We had a blast! Tom is very artistic and they shaved the breast cancer ribbon on the back of my head and then colored it pink with a highlighter. We then went out to the Harley-Davidson store in town and they bought me a couple of "Do-rags." The next morning we all went to church and I wore one of my new "head covers." My parents hadn't seen me bald yet and I waited until the service was over and I took off the do-rag and proudly walked out of the church. At first I thought my parents were going to faint, but I think that they were proud, too.

I never wore a wig because I just knew that it would fall off, get rolled up in my car window or be on backwards or something. I rarely wore anything on my head. If people didn't like it, too bad. Again, this is what it was. I actually washed my hair every day and put a towel on my head like I did when I had hair.

I was pretty up-beat and positive in the very beginning of this journey -- until I began chemotherapy. While I was on my way to my second treatment I told my roommate to turn around and take me back home. I just couldn't put myself through another treatment. If this was how I felt after only one, I couldn't imagine having to go through seven more. I called my mom and told her that I didn't want to have any more treatments; I didn't think I could handle it. It was at that time when she said, "You have to keep going, no matter how bad things get. You have to save yourself. It's up to you if you're going to beat this. Think of Cody and Sue and of us, we're not ready to lose you. God doesn't give you anything that you can't handle." Tammy wasn't going to turn around anyhow, so I went.

I became very discouraged because I felt like such a wimp. It seemed as if all of the older people who were going through chemo had an easier time of it then me. They would be pushing their IV poles around and eating treats that someone had made and brought in. All I could do was sit there. Food was the farthest thing from my mind. One day after a treatment I didn't even make it to the elevator and I had to turn around and go back. I was bawling my head off. Two of my oncology nurses explained to me that it's the younger people who have a hard time. Eventually it got to where I could eat some soup, but that was only because I knew that I needed something. My oncology team is remarkable. My chemo oncologist, Dr. Gene, was very thorough with his explanations about what I was going to experience.

My mom wanted to come up and help me during the chemotherapy, but Tammy thought that it would be easier on my family if they didn't have to see me like that. I was a complete wreck. During my first four treatments I was extremely nauseous. All I could manage to do was to crawl from my bed to the couch. I had my treatments on Thursdays, and I would be good until about four o'clock Saturday afternoon, and then it all went quickly downhill.

Eventually the chemo started "messing with my head." I got "chemo-brain." For the first 40 or so hours I would do crazy things. One night at about 11 o'clock I decided to bring one of my horses in the house – I thought that since I knew where Bubba lives then he should know where I live. He walked right in after me and we went into the kitchen where I gave him some horse biscuits. We then opened the refrigerator and Bubba, I and the three dogs all had our heads in there looking for some more snacks. The dogs shared a hot dog and Bubba got an apple. After that I brought him back outside and put him back in the barn. I called work and told them what I had just done, and they all knew then that I really was crazy.

One night I was actually out mowing the lawn until about 3:30 a.m. I had discovered that the old riding lawn mower had lights on it and they worked! I just couldn't seem to get myself off of that lawn mower. It was a good thing that we lived out in the country, so the neighbors never really knew what was going on.

Because it was summer, I called my friend, Guy Dutcher, who at that time was the District Attorney for Waushara County, and asked him if I had to wear a shirt while I was out and about. My logic was that if I didn't have any boobs, then how could it be indecent? He thought for a moment and then said, "No, I don't think that would be a very good idea."

Shortly after this happened, I attended my first Relay for Life. I went to pick up my survivor T-shirt and they gave me a cassette tape with this awesome song that was written talking about why we walk, why we do this. It never really occurred to me until I was there picking up my own T-shirt and listening to this song that the guy singing was talking about me. I was in such a state of crying when I got home. My sister, brother-in-law, and nephew were there and asked what was wrong. We listened to the tape and stood there on my front lawn sobbing. Then my roommate came up the driveway and asked what was wrong, did somebody die? Well – not yet.

When I went back that night to do the survivors walk I saw my name on one of the bags. To see that and to have that T-shirt with "survivor" on the back was one of the most intense -- almost like a slap-in-the-face -- moments of my life. No one ever thinks it's going to be them. I was the last person who ever thought they would have a name on a luminary in a Relay for Life – there was no breast cancer in my family.

At last year's Relay for Life I had been asked to do the survivor's speech. It hit close to home. The speech started out funny, and then at the end I had all the survivors stand up. Next I had everybody who had been touched by cancer stand up. Pretty soon everybody was standing. It may not have been politically correct, but I asked everybody to hold hands and say the *Lord's Prayer*. People were sobbing. This is how it is, this is how I live my life and it was very important to me that we collectively realize that God has something in store for all of us. It was my way of thanking Him for still being alive. The survivor lap was still hard. It's an experience I won't give up, but it's a very hard experience when you know that you are one of the people there with cancer that other people are trying to help. All these people are giving up their time, effort and money to help people like me. That was a moving part of my new life as a survivor.

One of my friends had 300 T-shirts printed up with "Kym Lindau Hope Fund" because I had my own separate savings account set up for that money. Out of the 300 shirts, we were only able to sell five. I gave a lot away including shirts to the whole confirmation class at my church. I left the room and when I came back in, they all had the shirts on, even the boys. They came up to me and said that they had all decided to wear them to school that Friday -- and they did. They don't know how much that meant to me. The impact that those kids had on me was monumental. Those are the kind of little things that keep me going and push the negative thoughts about giving up on life and letting everything go – it's the littlest tiny things that have actually helped keep me going. How selfish it would be of me to say I'm giving up.

People have to remind me sometimes that I'm not saving my life just for me, but for other people that I've touched and potentially can touch in the future. I would like to help them to get through the situation that I've gone through with having cancer.

I don't think about it every day, but each day I see the scars that go from the middle of my chest to touch my back on both sides. They are a reminder that I'm lucky I woke up this morning. I'm reminded of God's grace and the hope that LeRoy has put into my life. I believe this will open the doors to other women around the country who don't know where to go, don't know where to turn. Hopefully other people will take the baton that's passed to them and do what LeRoy's doing for us, because it's going to take more than just one person to help everybody that needs the help.

Two years later...

I myself thought after two years I would certainly be capable of returning to life as normal. But it doesn't work that way, my body doesn't work that way. I'm exhausted all the time; I have no energy the majority of the time. I experience bone pain so severe that some days I can barely stand, much less walk.

I was working against my doctor's wishes and pushing myself farther than I should have because I needed the insurance. So I continued to do what was expected of me at my job and knew that I couldn't quit. My health started to deteriorate even more than just because of the cancer. My doctors told me I needed to take time off and I needed to do it now. I went on short term disability and two weeks after that started I received a phone call and was told that there probably wouldn't be a job waiting for me when I came back. I am unable to work 12-hour nights, so even a casual position is unavailable.

This was right before Christmas and I was informed that my insurance would expire as of Dec. 31. At that point my world was already upside down and this shattered my hope. It was a real kick in the teeth. I had worked through the majority of my treatment and I had given everything I had to my job.

My mom and dad cashed in part of their life insurance policy to help me with bills. I get bills, two or three a day, every day. In October I wasn't able to come up with my half of the mortgage payment. My roommate sent in hers and it's sitting in an account somewhere, they won't take a partial payment. My house is now in foreclosure.

I don't have the money -- I don't have any money -- I spent the last of it on my medication. My eyes are all messed up from the chemotherapy and my teeth got pretty screwed up because of that too. It's things like that, plus my truck sitting in the shop because it needs repairs on it, those things have really impacted me. Farmers State Bank has been very good to me – LeRoy helped me get caught up, but I fell behind again and the bank is holding off repossession.

The doctor bills, the CT scans, the PET scans, the blood work, the medication – I'm in complete financial ruin. Before all this happened I had all my credit cards paid off and financially things were going in the right direction; I was done with school and was able to work more and do more things. Then I was diagnosed and pretty much from that day on, financially, I don't even see a light at the end of the tunnel.

The reality of my life is this -- do I pay my utility bill or do I buy my medication this week. It's a hard decision to have to make, especially during the winter. It would be different if I was unwilling to work, or if I was being lazy or out spending my money partying. Everything that I had worked so hard to achieve, such as trying to get myself set in a good financial position, was all gone in a matter of months. I didn't plan for the cancer to happen.

It's hard to hold your head up in a community when you're doing the best you can and then to lose your job and insurance on top of that. I've always been a giver and a caretaker and now I have to ask for help and it's really hard. And I probably don't ask for help as often as I should, I'm uncomfortable. Without the people who slip me $20 bills in church, or the secretary who calls me and says to come down and pick up some food, I probably wouldn't eat.

I'm still trying to be hopeful, but it's hard when people are calling you day and night. It's not a life that I would wish on anyone. It's not right, it's not fair, but I'm doing the best I can.

Lastly, I would like to thank LeRoy and the LeRoy Butler Foundation, the members of the Lutheran church, my family and friends for helping me, for giving me hope when I had none. I would also like to thank special friends Lynn Guiliani, Jeri Bye and Tammy Gee for sticking by me through all of this. Without the help from all these people, I don't think I would have made it this far!

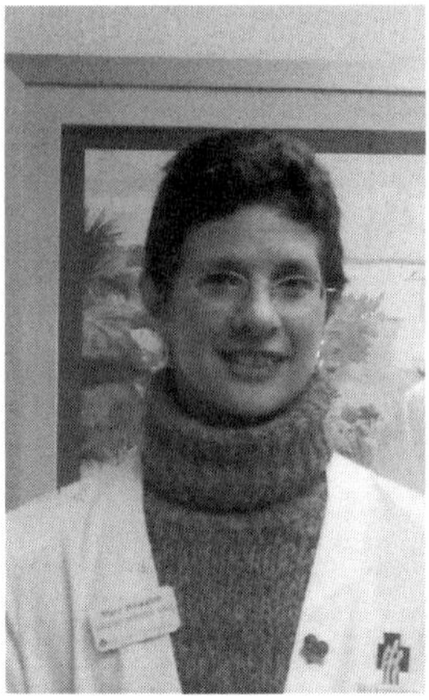

Chapter Five

The Love of God Through the Heartache of Cancer.
By Mary Kowatch, Wausau, WI.

I always tell people how God put me in the right place at the right time. As you will read, it would be hard to disagree. This is how I know that this is God watching out for my best interests.

I know that God is Holy and can not tolerate any sin in His presence. I would have to be completely perfect to go to heaven. That excludes me. But because God is love, He provided a way for me to know Him. That is through Jesus Christ. He died on the cross, rose from the dead and by doing this paid the penalty for my sin. The Bible says that if we accept this gift, we are then clothed in His righteousness, which is perfect, and not our filthy rags, as it states in Isaiah. Even though I was a young child, I knew enough that I needed to, by faith, place my trust in Jesus alone for my salvation and not rely on anything that I could do. I prayed that God would forgive my sins and asked Jesus to be my Savior. Because of this simple yet committed faith, I know that, as it states in Romans 8:28, "And we know that God causes all things to work together for good to those who love God, to those who are called according to His purpose."

This is why, even though I have shed many tears, and did experience fears, that I can still trust God with my future, no matter what the outcome.

Due to some financial needs in the spring of 2003, I started to look in the want ads for that perfect job that would fit into our family's lifestyle, as well as pay off a few bills. Although I'm a Registered Nurse, I had been a stay at home mom with our five children for the past eight years. Craig, my husband, had lost his job a year earlier and even though he was presently working, we were still financially recovering from that time in our lives. Thank God we experienced this "financial need." It played an important role in my outcome as you will see.

I always wanted a job in research and there it was in the paper, a 20 hour a week research job for an RN here in Wausau, Wis. It was in oncology, and though I had no background in cancer, I thought to myself this sounds very interesting. I talked it over with Craig, and sent in my resume.

I was called in for an interview. I was surprised at how well it went and how I was able to "sell myself" for the job. Usually I have a very hard time presenting myself in front of people. To my astonishment they hired me and I was to start in a few weeks. Later I was to find out from my manager that they had hired me over an oncology nurse that had applied for the position. They liked that I had shown from past experiences that I could work on my own. For the past six years I had volunteered at a Bible camp as the camp nurse where I was the only medical personal for a week or two at a time, 24 hours a day, seven days a week. It was often exhausting work, but I believe this was one of the main factors in my getting this research job.

Just three days after I started my new job, I had to have my gallbladder out. That went fairly well. Then within a month I found a lump in my right breast. A year and a half earlier I had a lumpectomy that was benign, so I watched it for a month to see if it went away with one of my menstrual cycles. It didn't. I had a mammogram in which the one centimeter lump did not show up, so they did an ultrasound next. The technician went and got the radiologist. He came in and finished the ultrasound himself, asked how old I was and told me he was sorry. I thought to myself, "That doesn't sound good."

I went in to have a lumpectomy the next week. While still in the operating room just after the lumpectomy was finished, I was awake enough to hear my surgeon gasp on the phone as pathology was telling her that the lump was cancerous, grade II-III invasive, a potentially fast growing kind. The surgeon came in and told Craig it didn't look good and left. Later she came back in the recovery room and told the both of us that the lump was cancerous. I remember not being surprised, nor did I cry. Before the surgery I had asked about how they preserved the tissue in case I wanted to be in a study. I felt God had prepared my heart to hear this news. We set up an appointment for more extensive surgery a week later, where my surgeon would take out more of the surrounding tissue, as well as sample a few lymph nodes to see if the cancer had spread. This is called breast conserving surgery with a sentinel lymph nodal biopsy.

Only a few people at work knew of my lumpectomy, and I didn't miss a day of work during this time. I told one of the oncologists, Dr. Steven Sorscher, who I worked with, and who ended up being my oncologist, that I was now looking for an oncologist myself. He turned on a dime from what he was doing and gave me a half hour of his time right then and there. He had been at the clinic for less than a year, and one of his specialties was breast cancer.

The next surgery, breast conservation surgery, and lymph node biopsy went fine. I had clear margins as well as negative lymph nodes and estrogen and progesterone receptor positive, which is a good thing. Being estrogen and progesterone positive means that the tumor fed off the hormones estrogen and progesterone and I could take anti-hormonal drugs after my chemotherapy to help prevent a reoccurrence of my breast cancer. My surgeon left for vacation the day after my surgery, which was July 3rd, so I had my follow-up appointment with one of her partners.

In the meantime at work, two oncology magazines had come out with articles in bold print on their covers about breast MRI's. I had never heard of a breast MRI, but it told about how much more a breast MRI could see versus a mammogram. I thought to myself, this sounds like something I need. Had I not had my job, I would have never known to ask for this test. I had to bring it up to four different doctors, but finally got one ordered. At first my oncologist said he would order it as a follow-up after my chemotherapy. But I came back to him a few days later and asked to have it as soon as possible to give me reassurance that there wasn't any cancer in the same breast, or the other one. He ordered it for me and said that most other doctors would not have done so (based upon the limited studies available at that time on breast MRI).

The main article I saw was from the *Oncology News International* magazine (July 2003, volume 12, number 7, page 24) regarding a study comparing MRI with mammography and ultrasound in a German study of 462 women with proven or suspected hereditary breast cancer.

The article quotes Dr. Kuhl as saying, "The first midterm results of this prospective clinical trial showed that MRI was more sensitive in detecting breast cancer than either of the other imaging modalities. MRI had a sensitivity of 95 percent vs. 34 percent for mammography and 42 percent for ultrasound. MRI depicted all but 2 of a total of 51 cancers detected in the study population, while mammography and ultrasound found less than half of the cancers."

By the time I had the test ordered I had started my chemotherapy. I was planning on losing my hair that I hadn't had professionally cut in 32 years. Earlier that year I thought about getting it cut, but thought God will let me know when it's time. It was time. I cried off and on for the two weeks before I was to get it cut, but that morning I was almost excited. I told the hairstylist not to worry if I liked it or not because it would all fall out in a week or two anyway. I did like it very much.

Chemotherapy was tough. I had four rounds of AC, three weeks apart from each other. I would work Mondays through Thursday 20-24 hours a week and then have my chemotherapy on Thursday afternoon. I would often get IV's on Friday and then again on Monday, as I would get very dehydrated from not being able to take in much food or fluids. I had trouble even swallowing my own spit.

Usually, by the fourth day I could eat a small meal and almost a normal meal by the fifth day after my chemotherapy. Most women I've seen don't have it that bad, but a few of us do. When I try to describe to my co-workers what eating and drinking was like for me, I would say it's like someone setting a bowl full of worms in front of you and telling you to eat it. That's how food and water seemed to me. I also had just enough energy to work my hours and no more. Fortunately, meals were brought to us from people from our church and neighbors on weeks of my chemo. I also had dear friends that came over and cleaned my house on occasion. It's hard to open up your messy house and let others in but it had to be done. I found that learning to be vulnerable with my needs built stronger relationships in the end.

Two weeks after my first chemotherapy, I was given a free ticket to the Women of Faith Conference in Chicago and was invited to go along with a group of women from my church. I accepted. The day we were to leave for the conference I noticed my hair was starting to fall out. I packed a couple hats and a pair of scissors. I had also started listening to a CD by a Contemporary Christian band from Canada called Downhere, especially their song "Calmer of the Storm." I thought to myself that I would love to hear that sung in church and showed Pastor Roger Smith the CD, hoping he would have someone sing it sometime.

The trip down was awful. I felt terrible, and emotionally I just didn't feel up for this. My hair had just started to fall out the morning I was to leave for the weekend. While in line the next morning for the first session, I was pulling out all the loose strands that were hanging down. A lady behind me, who wasn't with our group, said, "If you don't touch it, it won't fall out as much." She said she was an oncology nurse. I thought how like God to provide an oncology nurse to provide comfort to me during my first round of chemotherapy. Later that day, during our lunch hour, I lost track of my group but ran into these two women that were behind me in line that morning, one being the oncology nurse. I sat and had lunch with them. Hair was getting in my mouth, as it was windy outside, and was getting to be quite messy. I said to the two women, "Of all these women, there has to be a hairstylist in this group that could help me with my hair." Even though it was much shorter now it was still quite messy. The two women looked at each other and the other one, who wasn't the oncology nurse, said, "I'm a hairstylist." Even though I made it through the weekend without cutting my hair further, God had placed in my path both an oncology nurse and hair stylist for my support.

I now had my breast MRI and it showed two other spots of cancer in the same breast that was missed by breast exams from five specialists, a mammogram and ultrasound. It was decided that I would finish my chemotherapy and then have a mastectomy. Even though no cancer showed up in the other breast, I decided to have them both removed, as I thought screening for cancer in the other breast would be a problem in the future.

I might add here that there are some circumstances where mammograms can pick up things that a breast MRI does not. But I tell women all the time to get a copy of your mammogram report and read it. If it states that you have dense breast tissue and that no evidence of cancer is seen, it doesn't mean that you can be assured that there is no cancer. It is like if there is dense fog and someone was to tell you that they don't see any oncoming traffic, it doesn't mean that there aren't any cars coming. It just means they can't see any cars coming. This is the same thing with dense breast tissue. They can't see any cancer there and it doesn't mean that it is not! Especially if you have a lump that did not show up on mammogram in the first place. You want to make sure there is nothing else there that is being missed. I wish my doctors would have thought of that and saved me a couple of extra surgeries, but at least God put me in the right place where I would learn to ask for the MRI I needed!

I was dreading this next operation. Then I learned that the group Downhere was coming to Wausau, Wis. and the date of their concert was the night before my surgery. It reminded me of the time five years earlier, almost to the day, that Craig and I had hired a harpist to go to his mother's house to play her favorite hymns the night before her first chemotherapy to calm her spirit. I also learned that the radio station was giving away tickets to this concert. I told God that I wouldn't have time to listen to the radio to play their quizzes in giving away free tickets all week except for Friday afternoon.

Money was a bit tight, so it would have been a great help to get them for free. Also, God's best gifts are always free.

I remembered to turn on the radio that Friday afternoon. This was the last opportunity to win free tickets to the Downhere concert. The contest was still going and I heard the question to call in and win the tickets. I called, miraculously no busy signal. I was the first caller. I couldn't remember the answer so guessed. Wrong. I prayed for another chance. While dialing I knew to look to the end of Deuteronomy -- I found it. Once again, no busy signal and I was able to give the right answer. I had won two free tickets. And not only were they coming to Wausau, Wis., but to our home church. Even though our home church wasn't sponsoring the concert, the radio station had asked to have it at our church because of the larger auditorium it had. It was truly a personally wrapped present from God to me, as I had something pleasant to look forward to besides my surgery.

Craig and I got there a little early. I asked one of the sound technicians if they were going to play "Calmer of the Storm." He said a matter of fact they were and they had just added it back to their repertoire two nights ago, as it had not been played for the past six months. Later I got my picture taken with the band and shared with them what God had been doing in my life and what a gift of encouragement their concert had been for me.

That night after the concert I went home and had a peaceful night's rest. Very early the next morning Craig and I went to the hospital and Pastor Jon Payne met us there and prayed with us. I was also able to share with several of the nurses how God had blessed me so much during this whole time.

God is still blessing me tremendously. "Blessed be His Name. He Gives and takes away, my heart will choose to say, LORD, Blessed be Your Name." (Song by Matt and Beth Redman.)

Because of my new body image and not having reconstruction so I could detect any new cancers easier, my one prayer request that I did have back in January and February was that it would be a cooler than usual spring and summer, so that I could feel comfortable wearing layers of clothes if I chose to. (I also chose not to wear prosthetics as I find them uncomfortable. At first I thought everyone would notice my flat chest but I find they usually don't and it doesn't matter to me now anyway. Craig, my husband, was very supportive of my decision not to have reconstruction. In fact, he didn't want me to go through more surgeries and put myself at more risk just for the purpose of having breasts.) The summer of 2004 was an exceptionally cool summer. I don't believe we reached the 90's all summer. And the week I volunteered to be the camp nurse at Lake Ellen Bible Camp, we even had some nights in the 30's with record lows.

Speaking of Lake Ellen Bible Camp, for the past six years or so I have volunteered one to three weeks a summer as camp nurse, except the summer of 2003 while I was having surgeries and chemotherapy.

The camp had called in late spring of 2004 to see if I could be a camp nurse for a week or two that summer. At the time they asked I was quite a few months out from my chemotherapy, but I was still experiencing quite a bit of fatigue, so I said I didn't think I would be able to. The person who was in charge of getting the nurses for the summer never got that message. As a family, we decided to take the week of the 4th of July off and spend some time at my parent's cabin. I had taken that week off from work and was starting to get all the things packed that Thursday evening. Friday morning I was pretty well set when I received a call from Lake Ellen saying they were in desperate need of a nurse for that Sunday, and for the rest of that week.

I remembered in years past the enormous amount of flies and mosquitoes. It was almost like a plague, especially by the nurse's quarters. I literally killed hundreds of flies around the nurse's quarters in 20 minutes.

I was concerned about the potential risk of lymphedema developing in my arm if I were to get an infected bug bite. Since I had some lymph nodes removed from my right arm, I have to be extra careful not to get any cuts or scratches on it since even the smallest cut or bite can lead to lifelong swelling of that arm. I called my oncologist and asked him what were the risks, and he recommended that I should pass on the opportunity. However, since I already had made plans to have the week off and I was already packed to go, I accepted. Craig would bring the three older kids to his mother in Traverse City, Mich. for a visit, I would bring the two younger ones with me to camp and Craig would get some work done he needed to do.

That week was an unusually small camper week of only 60 campers and about 20 staff. I had time for naps when I needed one. (It often takes a full year or more to regain your pre-chemo energy level.) Also because of the unusually cool weather that week, I didn't see one fly for the first five days I was there and only a couple thereafter and very few mosquitoes. The warmest day was the last, Saturday, when Craig came up and we had time on the camp's beach and Lake Ellen all to ourselves.

There are always struggles in life (like when I was finally feeling like doing something fun with my youngest son in January of 2004 and took him out ice-skating and fell and broke my arm) but when you're able to give God praise and thanksgiving, He makes even the dark times be as the noon day sun. God is good! All the time! No matter what!

I ended up having a hysterectomy in the summer of 2005 for prophylactic reasons, to cut down on the estrogen my body was producing. I tested negative for the BRCA1 and BRCA2 genes, but that test can have a 10-12 percent false negative test. Also there might be other genes out there that are not yet discovered. If someone is BRCA1 and BRCA2 positive, they have up to a 60 percent chance of developing ovarian cancer as well.

I decided to quit my job in the fall of 2005. I was struggling emotionally having so many "cancer" issues in my life, my own health, the health of all the patients I worked with, as well as being a long distance support of 3-5 hours a week on the phone with Craig's mother who was battling end stage ovarian cancer. (My own mother was re-diagnosed with stage 4 breast cancer the summer of 2006 and my father has prostate cancer issues as well). After work I found myself in tears many times and I needed a few hours a day where I didn't have to think about cancer. We also decided to home school our children at this time due to some of our kids struggling in the public educational system.

Speaking of our kids, Nate, Beth, Abigail, Micah and Jonathan, who I enjoy and love more each day, they added humor to the time of the dark days of cancer in my life. They were ages 12,11,10,9 and 6 at the time of my diagnosis. Micah, our fourth grader at the time, came home from school and informed me that he learned that there were dinosaur bones, Allosauraus to be specific, in Wisconsin, where we live. He wanted to know if he could do some digging in our backyard to find some bones. I really didn't want to deal with all the dirt being tracked in my house and the backyard dug up, so I said no at first. The he asked to dig across the street in the park. I said you better stick to our yard and told him that I would need to call Digger's Hotline first to see if where he wanted to dig was OK. (Digger's Hotline has people come to your home and mark where all the power and gas lines are buried to prevent digging accidents.) I thought he would forget about it in a few days but he came home from school every day and asked if I had called yet. Finally I did. They asked me what the purpose of the dig was for and I heard a laugh as I told them, "So my son can find some dinosaur bones." They came out and marked our back yard and that same afternoon Micah was out there digging up a storm.

I had just finally trained our dog not to dig in the back yard -- until she saw the kids digging. Airedale Terriers are notorious diggers. It's like our dog thought, "Oh yeah, I remember digging, that's fun," and off she was digging too. I thought that there would only be about a two foot hole in this search for dinosaur bones, but that wasn't the case. Later that day, Craig came home from work to find barely the top of a head visible with dirt flying up from the shovel. At one time all five of our kids were in it digging away. This hole was about six feet wide and five feet deep.

My mother-in-law was on the phone with me while they were digging and asked how the kids were handling everything concerning me having cancer. I told her that they were doing fine. We calmly and openly shared all that I was going through, as well as God's provisions through it all. I told her that they were outside having a ball, digging this huge hole out in the backyard. She gasped as she exclaimed, *"WHAT?"* It then occurred to me what others might be thinking, especially our close neighbors who knew I was going through chemotherapy and whose kitchen window was 10 feet away and looked right over this big hole in our back yard. I reassured my mother-in-law that the kids weren't planning to bury me out in our back yard but were in search of dinosaur bones. Moral of the story is to enjoy a good laugh when it comes along, even if it's about cancer -- especially if it's about cancer.

I'm occasionally still called in by an oncologist or the American Cancer Society to talk with a new breast cancer patient, in which I am more than happy to do so.

Right after my case, my surgeon cancelled the digital mammography machine which was on order for the hospital where I had my surgery, and had a breast MRI machine ordered instead.

The competing hospital that was under construction and connected to the clinic where I worked also included one in their new diagnostic center. I encouraged them to put in a breast MRI machine to be competitive. I had to travel over an hour to have mine done, but now women in my community have two breast MRI machines available to them.

As an oncology research nurse, I had access to various oncologists that I sent e-mails promoting the breast MRI. I was able to go to a couple nation-wide oncology gatherings that some of the top oncology people in the country were at. I always made it a priority to make a beeline right for those people and ask about doing more studies with breast MRI. Especially doing MRI's with women that had a malignant lump that didn't show up on a mammogram – I tell them my story. There are many more areas of breast cancer that I feel needs more research done, and hopefully one day those will come about as well. I believe God is in charge of everything that happens in my life and I am responsible to be usable to Him to work all things together for the good, even if it means me having cancer.

Besides showing the awe striking love of God, I want women to feel comfortable in questioning their health care and be the managers of their health that they should be. Do your monthly self breast exams. It saved my life! Don't just rely on mammograms. Read your mammogram report. Be aware of what your body is telling you. Be aware of where God is leading you and give Him praise no matter where that path leads.

Only ten percent of all breast cancer is inherited, and 85-90 percent of all inherited breast and ovarian cancer are caused by BRCA1 or BRCA2 mutations.

- Christina Zaleski, MS, CGC, Senior Genetic Counselor, Marshfield Clinic, Wis.

"Calmer of the Storm"

Marc Martel/Jason Germain

When everything is wrong
The day has passed and nothing's done
And the whole world seems against me
When I'm rolling in my bed, there's a storm in my head
I'm afraid of sinking in despair.

CHORUS:

Teach me, Lord to have faith
In what you're bringing me will
Change my life and bring you glory &

There on the storm I am learning to let go
Of the will that I so long to control
There may I be in your arms eternally
I thank you, Lord, you are the calmer of the storm.

You rebuke the wind and the waves
Once again I find I'm amazed & the power of your will
Cuz I'm a child of little faith
I feel the wind and forget your grace
And you say, "Peace, be still."

There on the storm I am learning to let go
The white wave's high, it's crashing o'er the deck
And I don't know where I go
Where are you Lord, is my ship going down?
The mast is gone so throw the anchor
Should I jump and try to swim to land?

There on the storm, teach me God to understand
Of the Will that I just cannot control
There may I see all you love protecting me
I thank you Lord, you are the calmer of the storm.

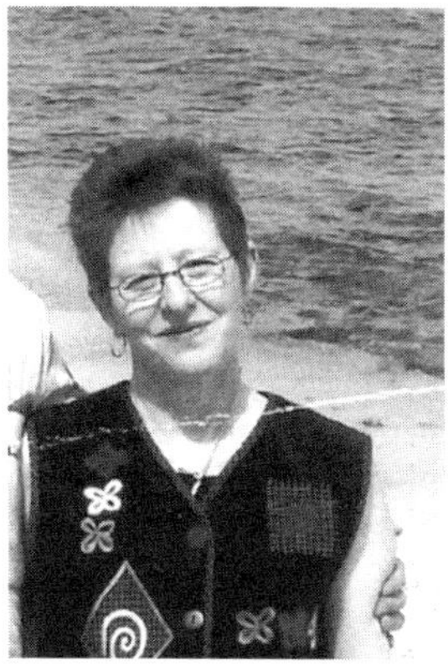

Chapter Six

God Grant Me the Serenity to Accept the Things I Cannot Change!

By Karen Marie Nelson, Wausau, Wis.

Throughout the course of my professional career, I had the opportunity to work extremely hard and "earn" my way into what traditionally would be considered "A Man's World." I sold insurance and financial planning services as well as started and ran my own Industrial Medicine Health Clinic in Wausau, Wis. for approximately 20 years. I was counted among the top producers in the life and health insurance industry. My husband and I had a beautiful $20,000 sunroom added on to our small house because I would be able to pay for it with my commissions from working in the insurance industry. Until…

Jan. 29, 2004 -- My first journal entry begins to tell the story of a learning opportunity I am still alive to speak and write about in January of 2007.

At 8:30 a.m. Wednesday, Jan. 7, 2004, I went to see a nurse practitioner in the gynecology department at our local health clinic. I had made an agreement with my (then) male business partner that if he would see his doctor regarding some major health issues of his own, that I would see my gynecologist in order to request medication to assist me with my crying jags and emotional upheavals. After all, I knew that I was right smack in the midst of menopause. And, isn't that word interesting? "Men A Pause."

I had been taking hormone replacement therapy (HRT) for approximately 12-15 years and had just (based on my own decision) weaned myself from them about 4-5 weeks prior. So, the nurse practitioner wrote a prescription for Zoloft a mild antidepressant to perhaps reduce the hot flashes. She wrote a prescription for yet another hormone replacement therapy for me to try. She also performed a breast exam and found nothing. She then scheduled me for my *ROUTINE* mammogram and blood work.

On Friday, Jan. 9, I showed up at the same clinic for my mammogram. Little did I know this would be the beginning of a new chapter and learning opportunity in my life.

The technician doing the mammogram kept calling me back into the x-ray room for more and more x-rays. I began to feel somewhat frightened but still fairly confident that all was well. And, would you believe that my boss's wife was waiting in the room for her mammogram to follow mine? All I could think about was that she would tell her husband that I may have breast cancer and that I might be unable to perform my job and therefore, lose my income which my spouse and I depended upon. After all, my husband had retired from teaching about three years before that date.

The final time I was beckoned back into the x-ray room, I was met by the radiologist. He told me that he saw a tumor on my left breast, and that it was necessary for me to immediately return to the OB-GYN department to meet again with the nurse practitioner whom I had seen just a few days previously.

When I saw the nurse practitioner, she immediately walked me to the surgery department at the clinic. I was then introduced to a general surgeon. I was alone at the appointment because I felt everything was routine. The surgeon showed me the x-rays of my left breast and did an exam of my breasts. He could not detect the tumor.

I had never met this man before. Consequently, I was not only uncomfortable but also frightened. The surgeon then told me that he would schedule a biopsy for me, but that I would have to wait because they only did the biopsies on certain days of the week and at certain times. So, I asked if I could get it done sooner in a town about one hour away and sure enough, I was scheduled for Wednesday, Jan. 14, 2004.

My husband, Gene, and I showed up for the biopsy at the appointed time and found ourselves in a large waiting room with many other women also waiting. I noticed that the women were "called in" three at a time. I felt as if I had never been treated in such an impersonal manner. It was clear to both my husband and myself that I was apparently viewed as just a number by the aides and technicians.

So, I got undressed, put my clothes in a bag and proceeded through the door pointed out to me. Two women then greeted me. The woman who was the doctor's assistant began explaining the biopsy procedure to me. She pointed out the table I would be laying on, the hole in the table my breast would be centered in, as well as the rest of the procedure. Now, I felt even more frightened. I had asked at the front desk if my husband could accompany me and I was given a flat "NO."

Next, I asked the assistant when I would get the results and she stated that it would be Thursday evening, Friday or the following Monday. I asked for a phone number so that if I did not hear by Friday morning, I could call so I would not have to go through *ANOTHER* weekend of not knowing. Her response to me was that if I was going to be that way about it, I for sure would not get the results until at least Monday or Tuesday.

It was then that I began to cry and sob. I felt as though I could not get through even one more minute of feeling ignored, uncertain, and afraid. It was at that exact moment when a most wonderful doctor arrived on the scene. He told his assistant to get my husband in the room with me. He then proceeded to tell me that he could do a procedure, where I would not be required to hang my boob in a hole on a long, flat, cold table. He also informed me that he was quite confident that if he did the procedure differently, that he would probably know whether or not the tumor was cancer in a few hours time.

Needless to say, we opted for the other procedure. (Why wouldn't we?) The doctor performed the biopsy while I was sitting up in a reclined chair. For the most part, it was painless. In about an hour, we met with the same doctor who had done the biopsy. The doctor so very gently informed us that the tumor in my left breast was cancer and that it would be necessary for me to have the tumor surgically removed as soon as possible.

It was at this point when we knew that it was necessary to inform my two adult children and my four grandchildren who lived in Milwaukee, Wis. Our friends accompanied us and we all went to dinner. Our friends took on the task of telling my kids about the diagnosis of breast cancer in my left breast, and the fact that I would be having surgery as soon as possible. I soon realized that my adult children would have preferred that my husband and I would have given them the news. In retrospect, I did not feel I had the emotional strength to tell my immediate family myself. I am the oldest of six farm kids and we lost one brother (only one year younger than myself) about 25 years ago. He was killed in a very bad car accident. I was afraid to tell my mother because I did not want to stress her with the possibility of losing another of her children. I phoned my youngest sister and asked her to inform my siblings and parents. Guess I was feeling very weak and vulnerable.

Now, we began a series of "quick" meetings with my gynecologist, my family physician, and two different surgeons. A friend of a friend of mine recommended a surgeon who only performed breast surgeries and who was very highly renowned throughout the United States. Just as a note, the surgeon was so highly qualified that he has since been hired away from that clinic and now manages a huge breast cancer clinic in the Eastern United States. We were able to schedule my first surgery for Friday, Jan. 23, 2004.

The plan was for the surgeon to remove the "sentinel" node from underneath my arm first and to send that to the lab for analysis for cancer. While that was being analyzed, he proceeded to remove not only one cancerous lump, but also two lumps from my left breast. The "sentinel" node came back from the lab positive for breast cancer. So, the surgeon then "harvested" 31 lymph nodes, which were all positive for breast cancer.

Within a very short time after the initial surgery was finished, I was awakened by the hospital staff and immediately put into a wheelchair and told that I was ready to be taken home. I was sitting in the wheelchair vomiting profusely. So, they actually did wait until I was done with that learning opportunity before they wheeled me out to the car.

About one day after the initial surgery, my surgeon phoned me and spoke with my daughter, Penny, and myself. He reiterated that the 31 lymph nodes and the two lumps in my left breast were Estrogen Positive, Stage III breast cancer. He also told me that it would be necessary to remove my left breast just as soon as possible in hopes of avoiding additional cancer. In retrospect, I wish that I had had both breasts removed at that time so that I might have avoided the constant threat of the cancer re-appearing in the other breast. My surgeon also told me very clearly that because the breast cancer was Stage III that the odds were that I would have a 20 percent chance of living for five years. He told me that he had one patient who had as many positive lymph nodes as I did who is still alive after 15 years. So, there was my hope, at least as far as my surgeon was concerned.

On Feb. 2, 2004, our friends, my daughter, Penny, and my husband accompanied me (once again) back to the hospital for more surgery. I showed my surgeon a copy of a medical study indicating that redheads have a much lower pain tolerance than people with less fair skin. We laughed and joked together about it; however, I was so frightened that I felt I had to make every point possible to assure my safety in and through this huge "learning opportunity."

Since I had learned a very tough lesson being sent home from the hospital within minutes after my first surgery, I convinced my surgeon that I should be allowed to stay over night at the hospital following the removal of my breast. Can you believe that? They gave me 200 milligrams of morphine every hour throughout the night. Great, then I could actually sleep.

On Feb. 3, my 55th birthday, I was released from the hospital. I was feeling many feelings of anger, guilt and depression. My husband, daughter and friends were instructed on how to empty all the drainage tubes and change the dressings. Oh, I was so excited. What a way to celebrate my birthday.

The cards, flowers and food began to arrive at our house. We were very grateful as both my spouse, and certainly not myself, were in a physical or mental frame of mind to actually do much of anything ourselves.

We moved my husband's recliner out to our new sunroom and that is where I virtually lived for several months. It soon became clear to me that not only my immediate family but my extended family (living all over the entire country) began putting my name on prayer lists so that I was being prayed for literally all over the world.

Now, it is time to tell you about my learning opportunities with chemotherapy and radiation. Before they could begin administering the chemo, several tests had to be completed. They began by doing a PET scan, which was to search for the possibility of additional cancer in my body. The PET scan took more than four hours because first they injected some radioactive material into an additional IV besides the porta-catheter that was already placed in my right breast. So, that meant an additional "poke." Then I was instructed to lay flat and quiet for one hour. They then performed the scan itself, which took another hour. They wheeled me in a wheelchair outdoors to a truck where the scanning machine was located. Once again, I felt cold and frightened. I certainly did not care for the large machine. There was very little room between my head and the top of the machine. The technicians wrapped my arms and legs tight to my body with some large bed sheets.

They took six sets of pictures and the so-called "camera" was over each area of my body for about ten minutes or so. The only really bad part was when the machine was directly over my head and I could not, of course, move. I am extremely claustrophobic.

Also, before chemo could begin, another very important test had to be performed. They drew some of my blood, added some radioactive material to it and then placed it back in my body. They had big overhead cameras that took pictures of my heart to help determine whether my heart would be strong enough for one certain kind of the chemo they would be giving me. The good in this test is that it only took about a half-hour.

Oh yes, they needed yet one more test before they would start administering the chemo. That test was a "simple" colonoscopy. I had to drink a gallon of banana-raspberry smoothie. It was during the time of drinking this wonderful smoothie that I looked at myself in the mirror. I could not believe how disproportionate I looked. I felt that both my scars and I looked like a "freak." It seemed like the saddest moment of my life. So, I said to myself, "Oh well, Karen, you must get used to it." Then I started to sob in spite of my attempt to cheer myself up. Little did I know and understand that there would be many more "sad" days.

I decided to visit my beautician for a "preliminary" hair cut before starting the chemotherapy. I talked with her about cancer, chemo, losing my hair and several other things that seemed to be bothering me. She was absolutely wonderful. She told me that when I started to lose my hair that I should call her; she would come to my home and shave my head. She knew that I would be less embarrassed at home and would not have to worry about walking into the beauty shop with lots of other women.

My surgeon recommended that I get myself a wig before my hair started to fall out. So, one of my daughters got me a red wig. During the course of my hair loss, I also acquired two other wigs. One was dishwater blonde and the other another shade of red. I actually liked the blonde one the best because then I was able to be "blonde" for the first time ever.

After only one dose of chemo, my hair was falling out in big clumps on my pillow. There were also tiny pieces of hair everywhere. I awoke one morning with little pieces of hair in my mouth and in my eyes. My scalp hurt a great deal and was very sore.

When I showered, more than just the water fell from my skin. I wrote my true feelings in my journal and I simply wrote, "I hate the whole damn thing." That night I prayed, "Dear Lord Jesus, please give me the strength and understanding to welcome my hair loss and to know that the chemo is doing its work." It hurt so much to look in the mirror and see big bald spots on my head. I called my beautician and scheduled an appointment for her to come to my house the following evening.

Early the morning of my first chemo treatment both of my young granddaughters, from Milwaukee, Wis. called me and told me what a good thing it was that I would be getting the medicine to make me better. They were three and five years old at the time. Both my granddaughters and my grandson (who was six at the time) tried on all of my wigs. They thought it was great fun.

I had been told that I would be given two rounds of chemo treatment. The first round was once every three weeks for three months and the second round was the same. The drugs were extremely strong and powerful (so I hoped anyhow). My first experience with chemo began with being given an anti-nausea pill (which by the way, did not work) and about five steroid pills. Then, the nurse "pushed" in the red medicine that was in a large long syringe. I was told she needed to "push" it so that she could watch closely while it went in, so she could be sure that none of my veins would burst. That in itself only took about 20 minutes. She used my porta-catheter. Then the second drug was given to me via a drip IV. That took about one hour.

The day after my second dose of chemo was very challenging for me. I began to vomit and vomit and then began to choke on the vomit. However, I kept telling myself that it was a good thing because the toxins were "coming out." Also, very soon after the second dose of the chemo, my mouth became filled with canker sores and my throat was white with bumps in it.

Here, I must talk more about my husband, Gene. Traditionally, Gene is very quiet and often struggles with finding the "right" words. I had been telling him about a friend who had told me to stop "whining" about the fact that I would be losing all of my hair. And, other women would always say things to me like "Don't worry, it will grow back." Well, guess what? Those words did not help at the time.

My husband gave me some great words of wisdom -- he simply said, "You thought in the beginning when you were told that you had breast cancer that you could not get through it. And, now you have adjusted to the idea and you are doing fine. You thought you could not get through the first surgery and you did just fine. You thought you could not get through having your breast removed and you did fine. You thought you could not get through the first session of the chemo and you have gotten through that. So you see, you can and will get through losing your hair."

I then looked at him through my tears and thanked him for his kind words. I also told him that moment, "As soon as we get through the chemo and radiation, we are going on the greatest trip we have ever been on." Needless to say, he agreed with me.

Another super important part of my "learning opportunity" has been to have faith in my God and in myself. I have always had what I felt was a lot of faith, however, it was nothing compared to what I feel now and the thankfulness that I feel because the good Lord lets me live each day as if it were my last. Every morning when I wake up, I begin the day with my "Thank You God" for letting me wake up well, prayers. I also have come to realize how important it is that *I S L O W D O W N* my entire life and career.

I came to realize that I had let "stress" rule my life. This brings me to my belief that, "What You Think About Is What You Are." I am also always working on the fact that I can change no one else but me. And, if I am not careful, it is possible for me to think myself right into the grave. I believe this can happen if I think I am so sick that I will not live and if I think about nothing but negative thoughts. I must believe that I can do what it takes to survive (With God's help as well as the love and prayers of those whom I surround myself with).

Right near the end of the chemotherapy, I went to the clinic and was fitted for a prosthesis to fill the area where my left breast was supposed to be. I cried a great deal and yet, at the same time, told myself how fortunate I was to be alive. Our health insurance company approves one pretend boob every four years. So, the technician informed me of the importance of always handling it with care. We did not want it to rip or tear. Then of course, I also had to be fitted for a special brasserie, which would hold the prosthesis in place. So, another "learning opportunity." Also, I managed to find a swimming suit equipped with special pockets on each side to hold the prosthesis.

About this time, we began to experience extra challenges with finances. I had always worked out of the home so now we were "missing" the great income I had been bringing into the household. A few years before the cancer diagnosis, my husband had retired from 34 years of teaching. However, he was substitute teaching every chance he got. But, the bills were still coming in. My hospital and clinic bills averaged $20,000 a month for several months. Luckily, we had reasonably good insurance through my husband's former employer. Speaking of bills; our local clinic actually turned us over to a collection agency when at one point our total was down to $500. I literally begged them, including their management people, to work with me but they said "absolutely not." So, now we have that on our credit rating. Incidentally, we did pay the $500, but we had to pay it to the collection agency.

After finishing the chemo treatments, it was time to begin radiation oncology. I was told that I would be receiving radiation every day for approximately eight weeks. I drove myself to the local radiation clinic and had to be measured for the upcoming procedures. I was very sad when they had me lay down on a very cold table and refused to even give me a sheet or blanket to cover myself with. I was still very uncomfortable about the appearance of my body with my left breast missing. The technicians and the oncologist spent several minutes moving me back and forth; up and down and then administering two "tattoos" so that they would always know how to position me. Neither the doctor nor the technicians bothered to talk or explain to me what they were doing. I started to cry and they simply proceeded as if nothing was wrong.

During the time of chemo and radiation, I also went every other day for physical therapy for my left arm. Lymphedema is a common side-effect from having had many lymph nodes removed. My understanding is that there will never be an active immune system in my left arm. What that means to me is that my arm does not want to move or stretch very well.

Finally, we were able to take the trip I felt that I had been keeping myself alive for. We took a week's vacation in Jamaica. It was so wonderful for us to relax together. We took lots of walks and simply enjoyed being together for a pleasant and welcome change. My spouse has been through hell and high water for me and I was so glad we could have this wonderful time together.

My doctors and oncologists schedule me every three months for ultrasounds, CT scans of my neck, chest and pelvis, as well as bone scans. About once every six months I receive PET scans. We also get my blood checked on a very regular basis due to a blood clot in my right arm.

In October of 2005, when I went through my "routine" scans and tests, the radiologist discovered a "different" swelling on the left side of my neck. My surgeon insisted that he do a biopsy in the area because it was something we had not seen on the tests before. In early November, my surgeon showed me the pathology report. He had removed cancerous tissue in my lower neck. The good in it is that the scar is sitting right in one of the wrinkles in my neck.

Both Gene and I were devastated. My oncologist told me it was just a matter of time before the cancer would spread throughout my entire body. He also told me that it was "essential" that I start chemotherapy as soon as possible. I scheduled myself to start the chemo on Jan. 2, 2006. Then I went home to pray.

It was during this time that I received a phone call from another very good friend. He and his wife had heard about the breast cancer in 2004, and he was simply calling to inquire about my health. So, I explained about the "new" diagnosis. This time it was classified as Stage IV metastatic breast cancer. Once it spreads to another part of the body, it is considered metastatic.

The same friend had told me previously about a good friend of his who was doing battle with breast cancer. Her name was Carol.

The above information is important because when I finished telling Jim about the re-occurrence, he asked me if I would mind if he gave my name and phone number to Carol and her husband. He informed me that she was involved with some program out of Ottawa, Canada and both she and her husband felt that between their faith in God and the Cancer Research Center in Ottawa, she was healthy and doing well.

Just a few days later, I received a phone call from Carol's husband. He told me many things about the Cancer Research Center and gave me the name and phone number of the doctor at the center. When I called and spoke with the doctor, I became very excited and hopeful. He told me it would not be necessary for me to travel to Canada. He explained that if I were to enter their program, it would be necessary for me to have my blood drawn at the local clinic. There it would be "spun" and the remaining plasma would be shipped to the center in Canada via FedEx overnight. He explained that the plasma would be analyzed for over 50 different markers and that he would then be able to determine whether or not I needed to start chemotherapy at this time. He informed me that the clinic would then prepare and ship to me, whatever compounds would be necessary based on my test results. He indicated that it would take about 12-18 months for me to complete the program.

This was pretty exciting to hear. However, there was only one huge problem. Usually, I consider things as challenges and not problems. But, this truly was a problem. He told me that the cost would be $6,000 for the first six months and then $4,000 every six months thereafter. Insurance does not pay for healthcare or medications coming from Canada. So, right at that exact minute, I made a major decision. I told the doctor that if he would "take my word for it" that I would somehow organize a "benefit" for myself in order to raise the money to pay for the program that just might save my life.

The first thing I did was to call my oncologist and inform him that, at least for now, I would not receive chemotherapy. My family members, my husband and myself felt that I was not yet strong enough to endure chemo at this time.

The rest of the story is incredible and wonderful. As I prayed, I received the name of a very special lady whom I had had the opportunity to do some professional work with about 10 years ago. I called her and she agreed to meet with me that same afternoon. Now I was really praying hard. What would I tell her? What would I ask her for? How would I ask for her help?

When we met, I told her my story about the re-occurrence of the breast cancer and my plan to have a "benefit" in order to raise the money to pay the clinic in Canada. She asked what I needed from her. I then told her how I had prayed all the way to her office for the right words to ask for the help my husband and I needed. The words suddenly started to flow from my mouth. I explained that we did not have a place to have the benefit. I also explained that it would be nice if we could have some music and some food.

She then, very matter of fact, told me that she and her husband could provide us with the place, with a band and even food. As you might imagine, I began to cry tears of thanksgiving and joy. She shared with me that she knew God must have sent me to her. I discovered later that her secretary had just recently passed away from breast cancer. I was told that this lady and her husband had literally taken care of their employee as she endured the complications of breast cancer. I did not know that before I went to see her. What a gift she was to me!

The Monday following the benefit, I mailed the signed contract and money off to the Cancer Research Center in Ottawa, Ontario, Canada. Praise God and friends and family.

It has now been three years since I was first diagnosed with breast cancer. Just two days ago, I received my latest report from the clinic in Canada. I am told that the most important factor, my immune system, has improved 600 percent since I started the program.

I believe that I am still alive today because it is God's plan for me to help other women and their families who have breast cancer. I am very happy and thankful and continue to thank God for every day I wake up well.

To find a genetic counselor in your area, go to www.nsgc.org, click on the link "Find A Genetic Counselor."

- Christina Zaleski, MS, CGC, Senior Genetic Counselor, Marshfield Clinic, Wis.

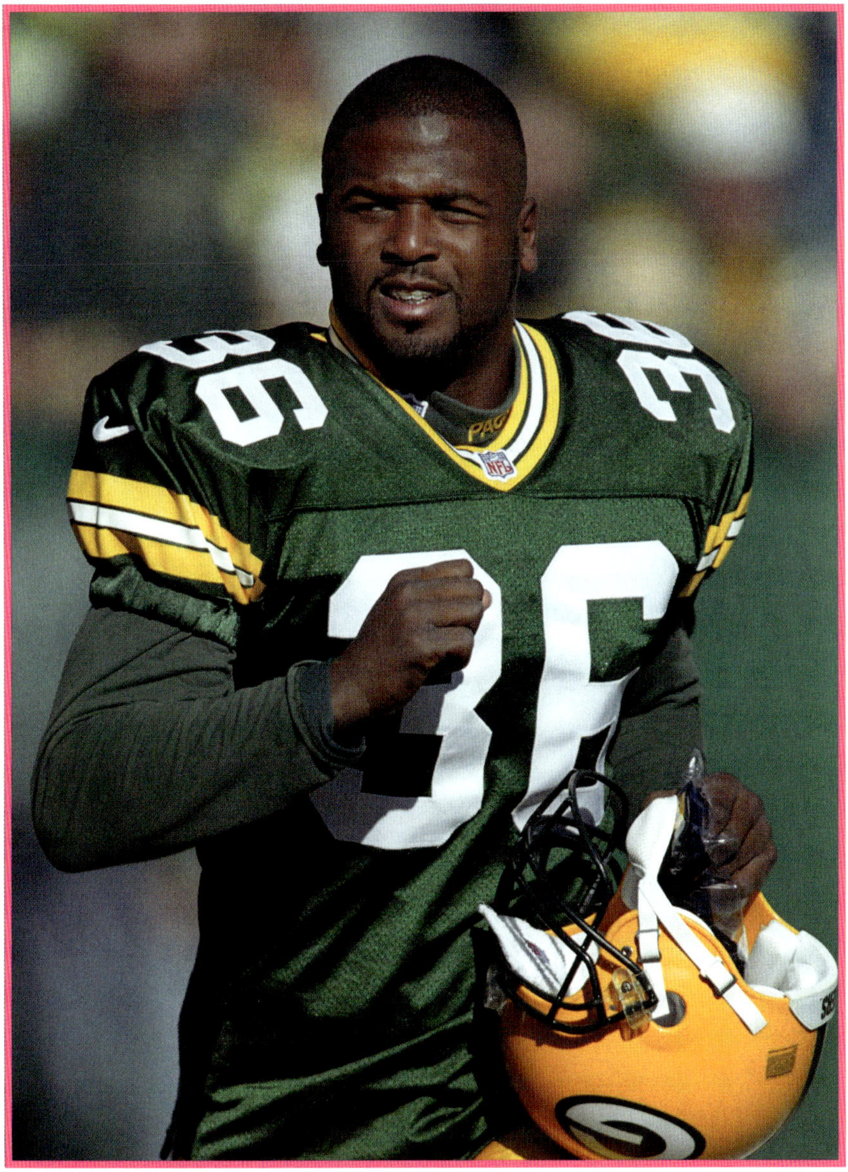

LeRoy Butler, a member of the Green Bay Packers Super Bowl XXXI championship team and creator of the Lambeau Leap, has turned his attention to the importance of raising awareness and funds for breast cancer survivors.

Photo by Mark A. Wallenfang

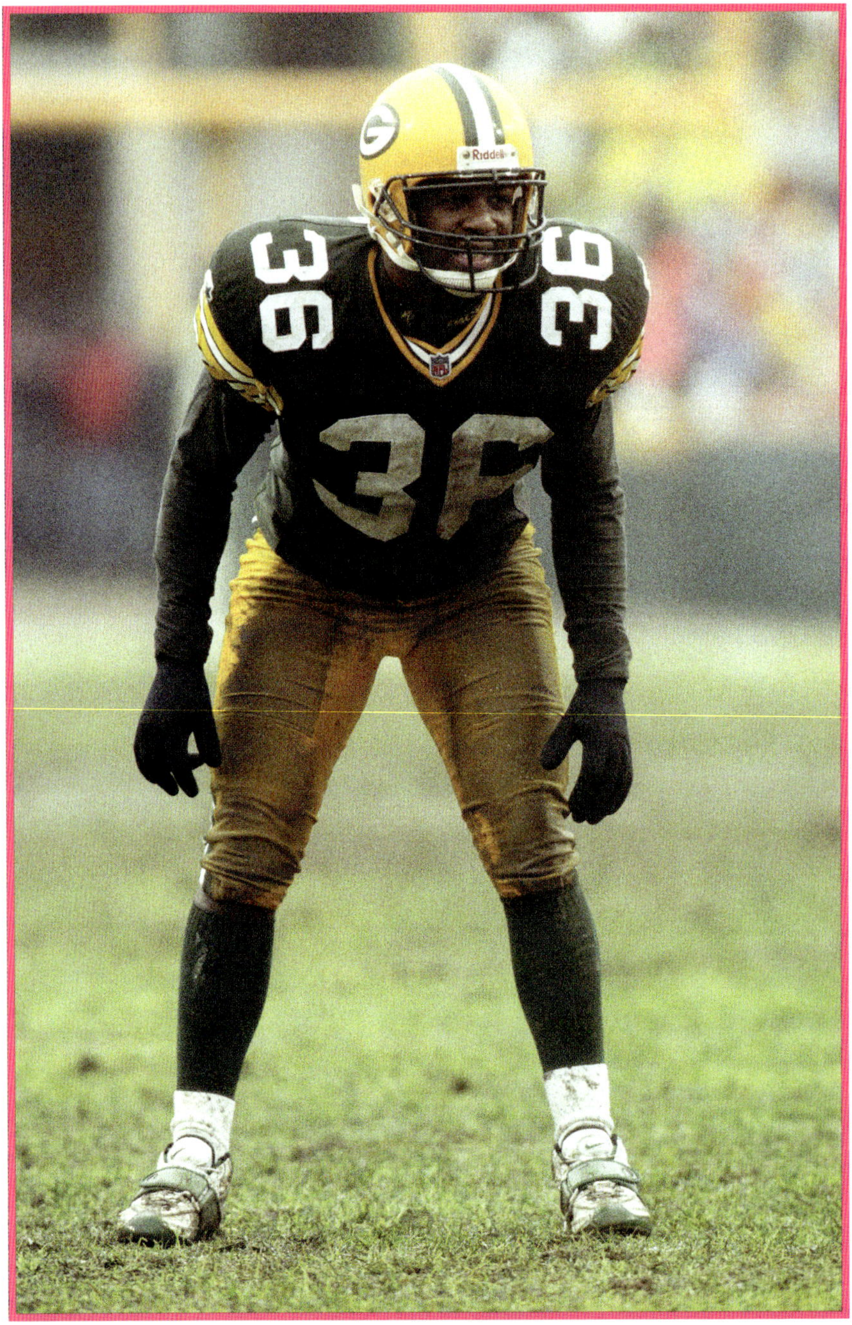

The January 1997 Green Bay Packers vs. San Francisco game where LeRoy Butler was first inspired to help women battling breast cancer.
Photo by Mark A. Wallenfang

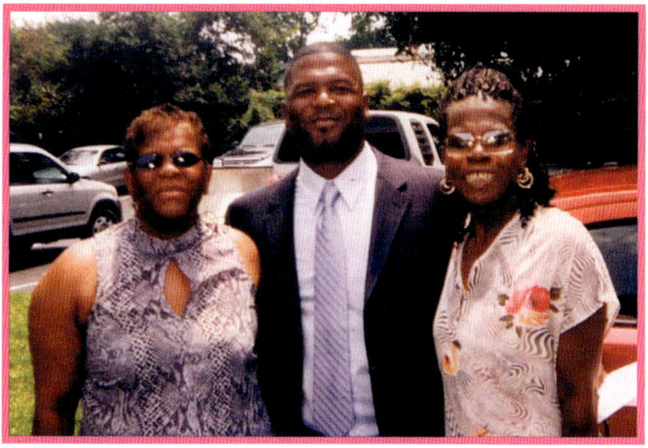

LeRoy Butler with two special women in his life, his mother, Eunice Butler, and sister, Vicki Wilson.

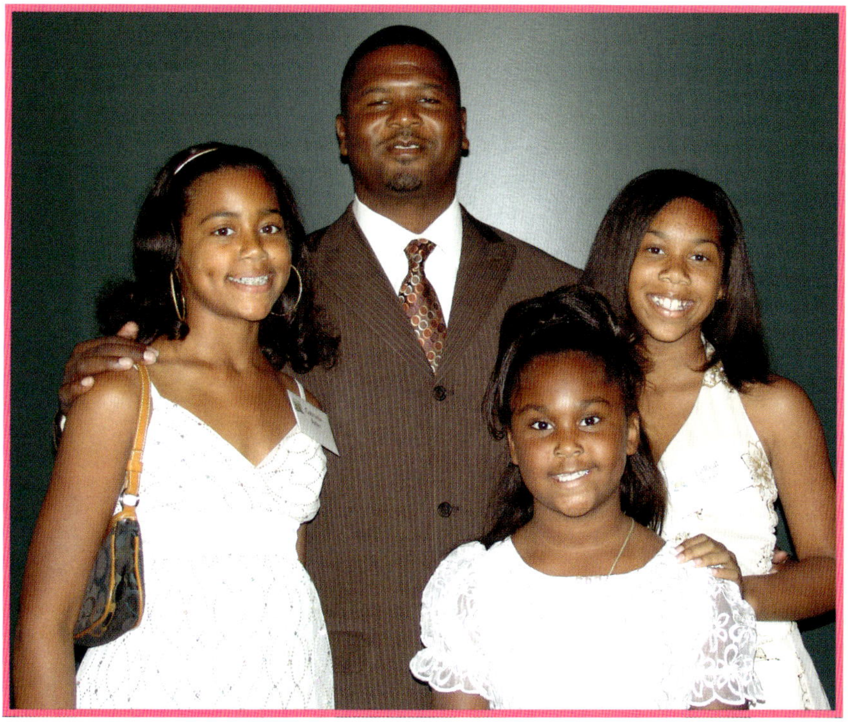

LeRoy Butler was inducted into the Green Bay Packer Hall of Fame in 2007. He is pictured at the induction ceremony with three of his daughters, LoReal, Gabrielle and Danielle. Not pictured is Sharon.
Photo by Rick Severson

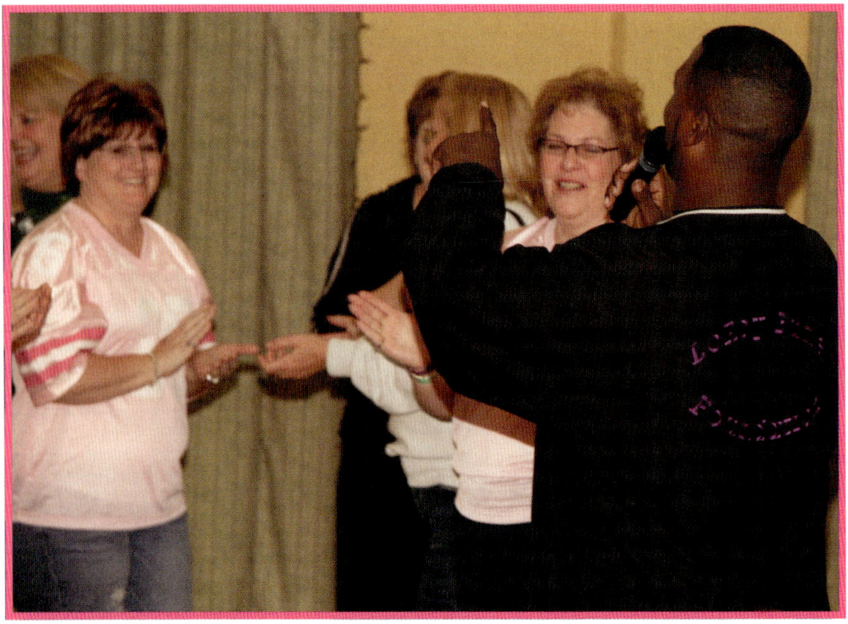

LeRoy Butler honors some of the breast cancer survivors who have been helped through his foundation during the LeRoy Butler Foundation Battle of the Borders event in December of 2006.
Photos by Bonnie Wood

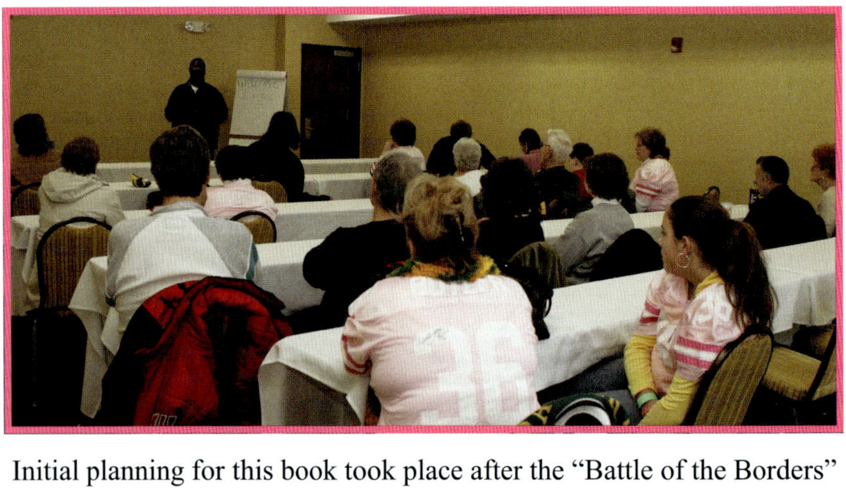

Initial planning for this book took place after the "Battle of the Borders" event, December 2006.

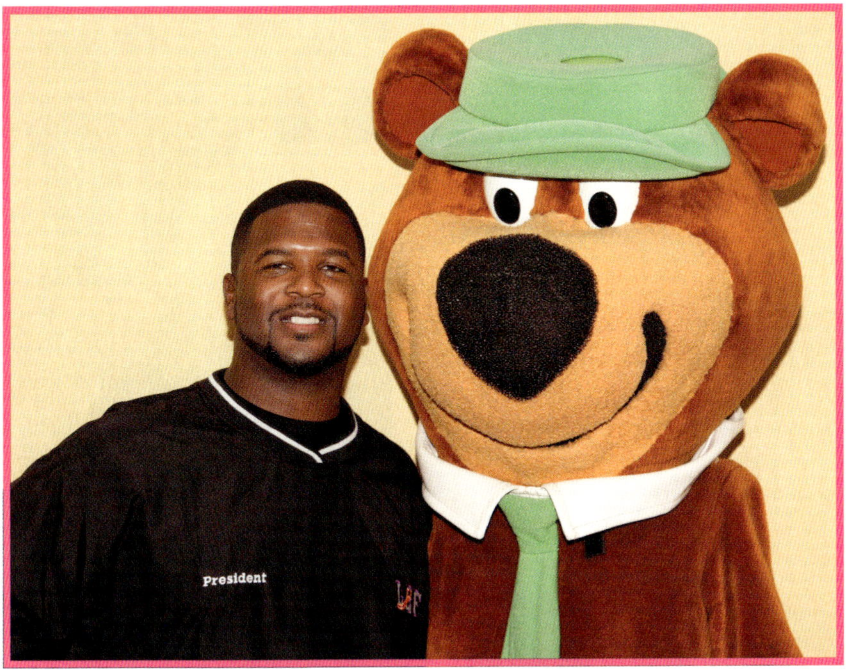

LeRoy Butler and Yogi Bear at Jellystone Park, Warrens, Wis.
Photos by Bonnie Wood

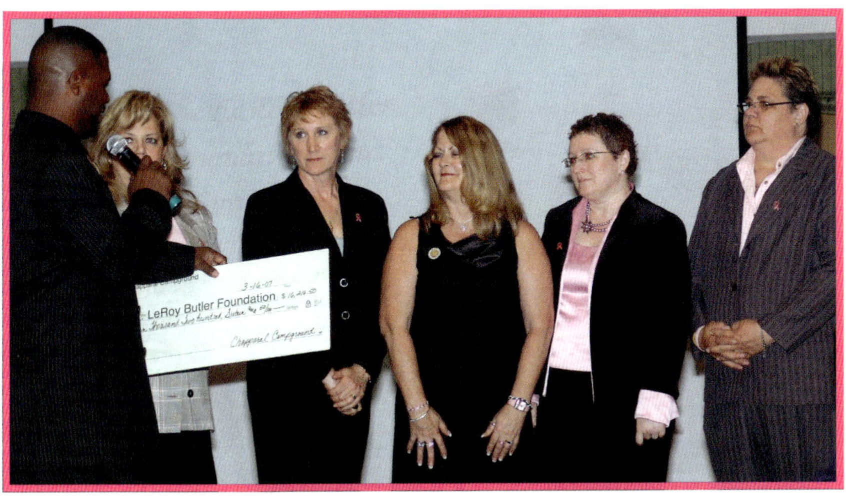

The LeRoy Butler Foundation has raised over $300,000 to help women with breast cancer. Check presentations took place at the April 2007 Spring Fling in Warrens, Wis.

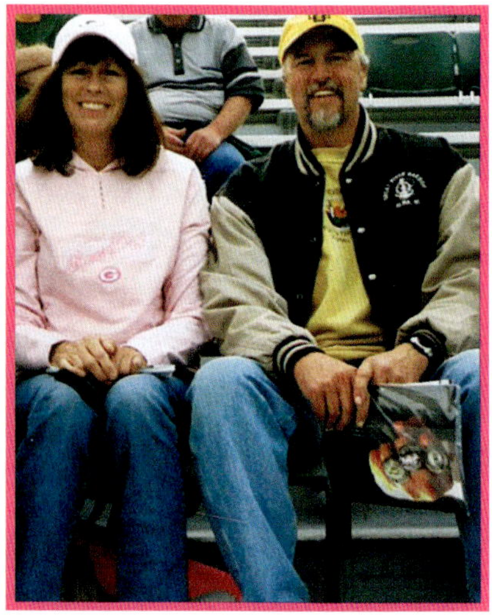

Janet Evans and her husband, Hale, at Lambeau Field, Green Bay, Wis. for a home opener honoring the Super Bowl XXXI team

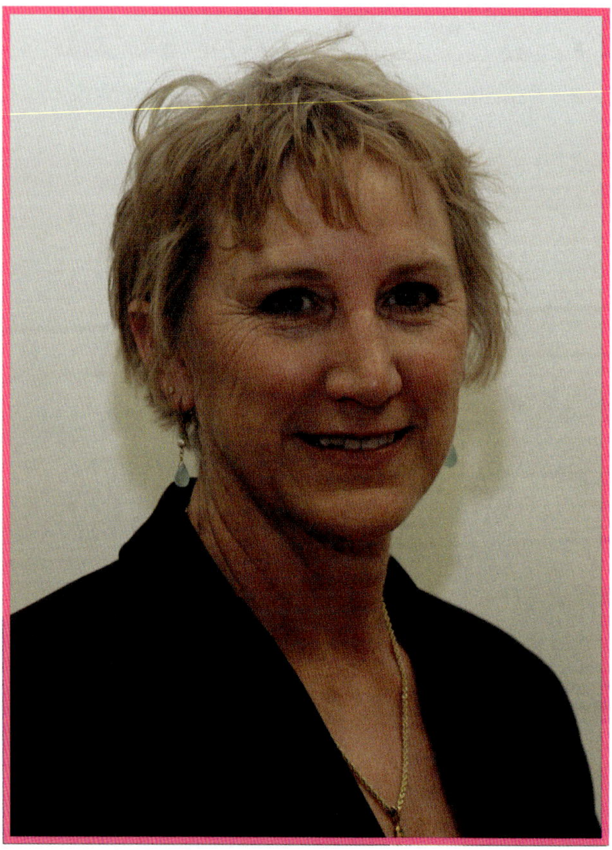

Ursula Koxlien at the LeRoy Butler Foundation Spring Fling, April 2007

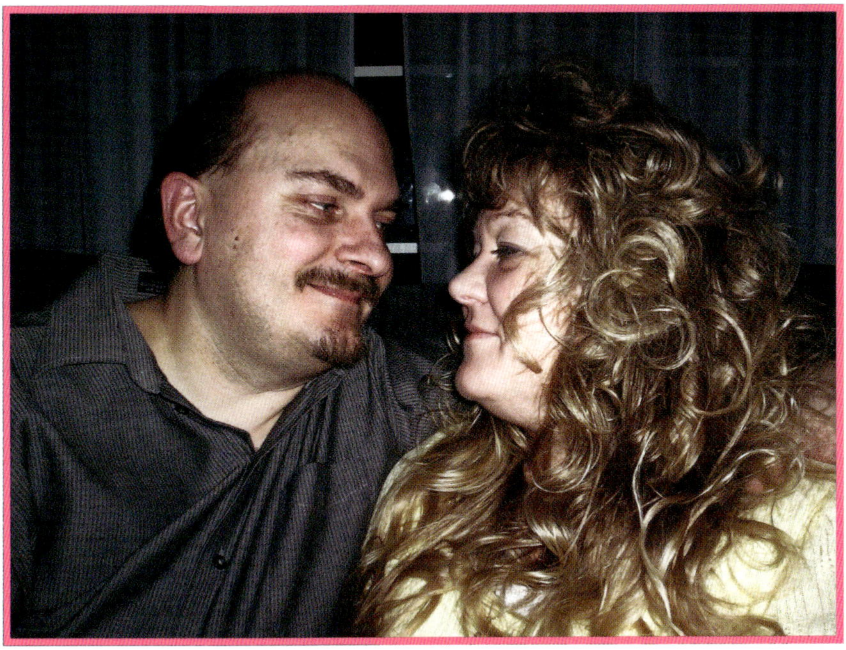

David and Tammy Oestreich

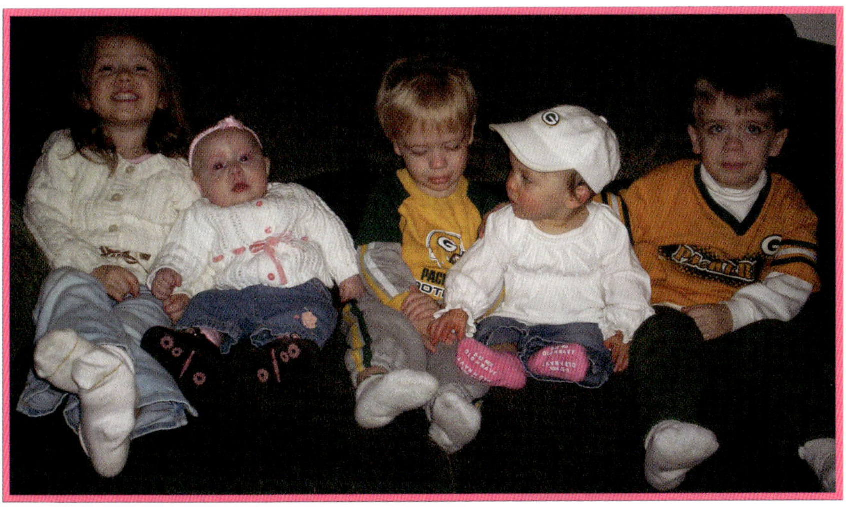

Tammy's daycare children and her hope for the future

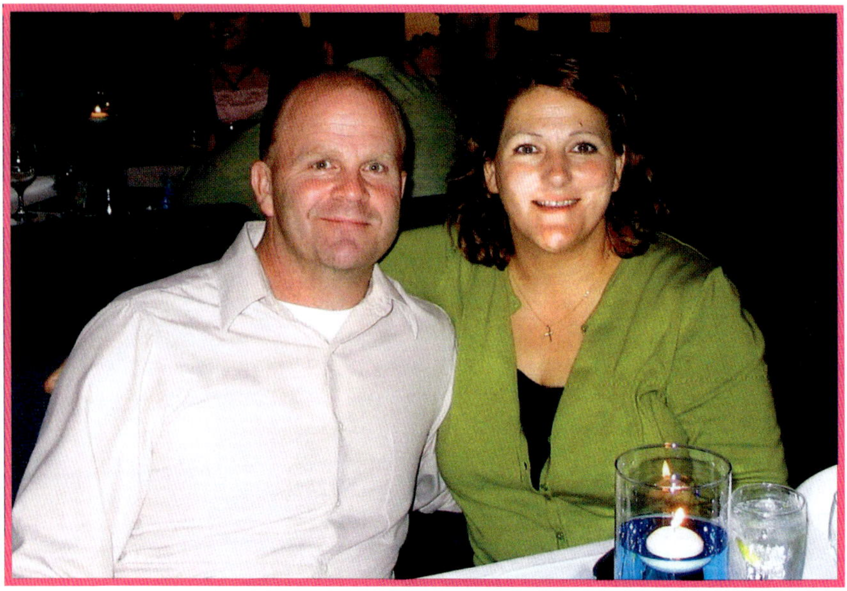

Stefka Meddaugh and her husband, Todd

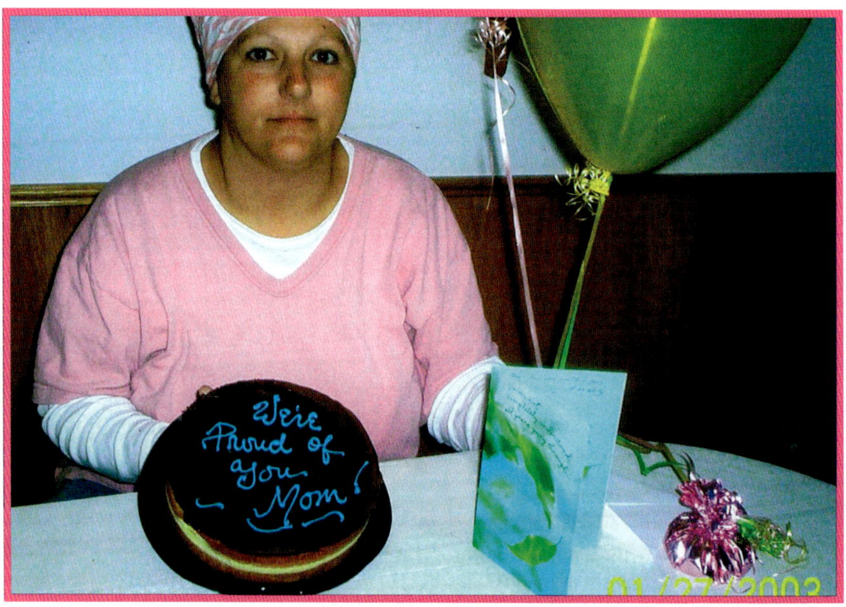

Last day of treatment – a celebration for Stefka and her family

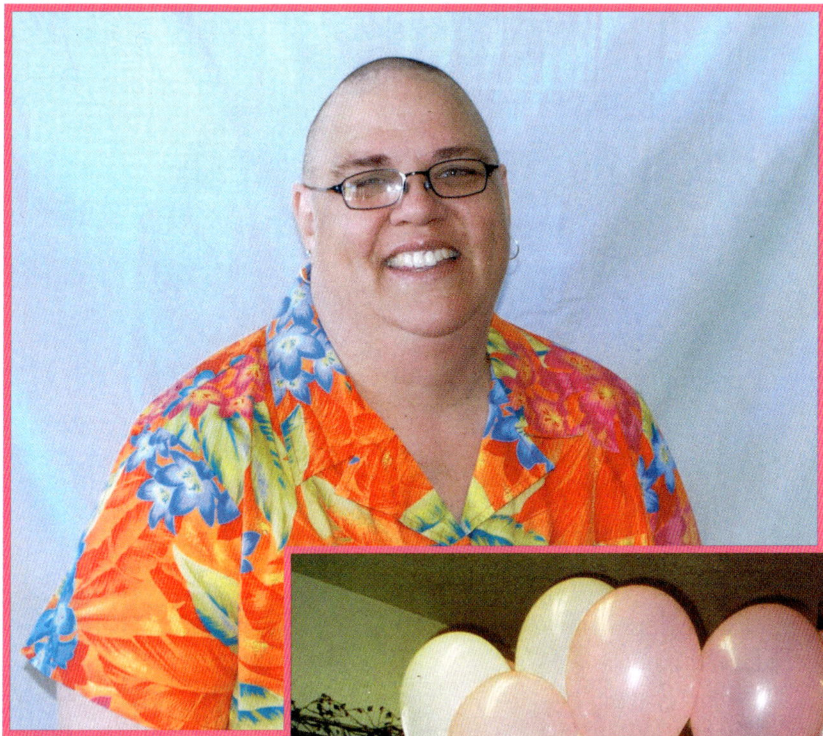

Kimberly Lindau, photo courtesy of Mary Kunasch – *Waushara Argus*

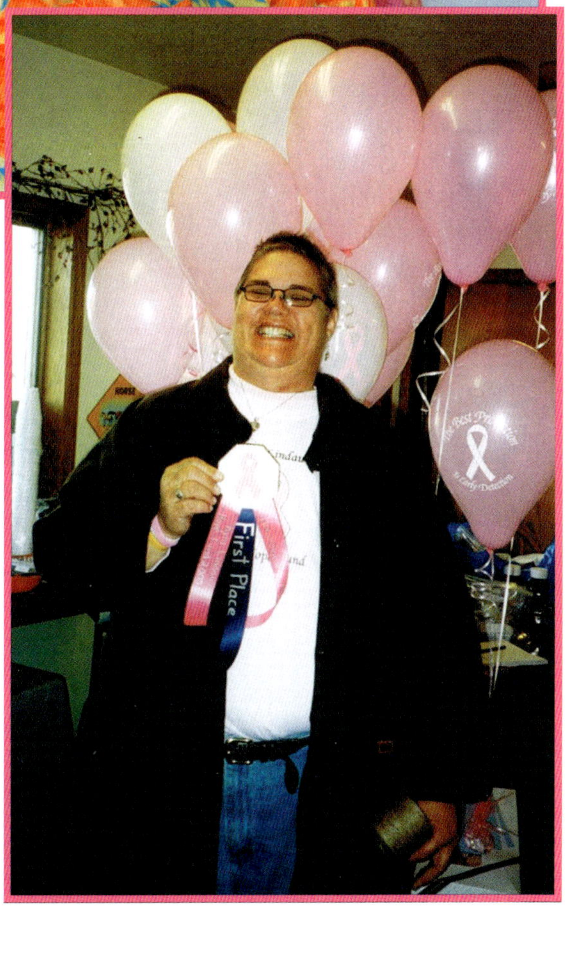

Kym at a Natural Horsemanship breast cancer fundraiser in her honor

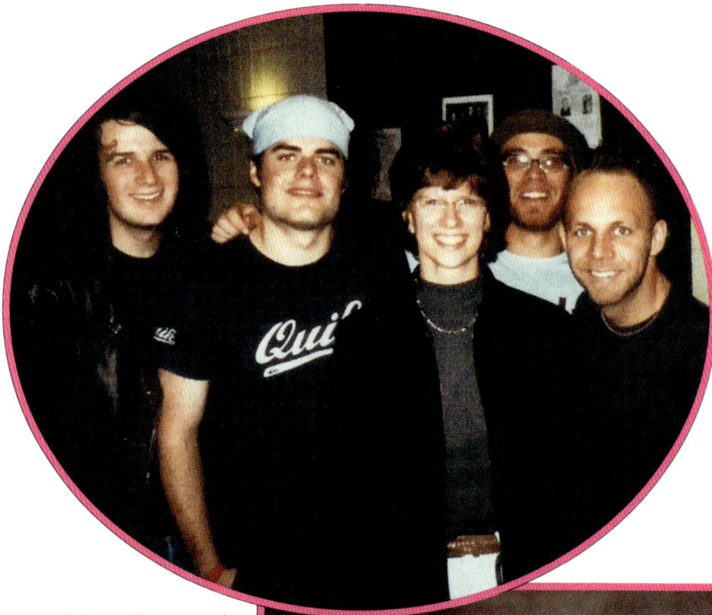

Mary Kowatch and the group, Downhere, at a Wausau, Wis. concert the night before her surgery

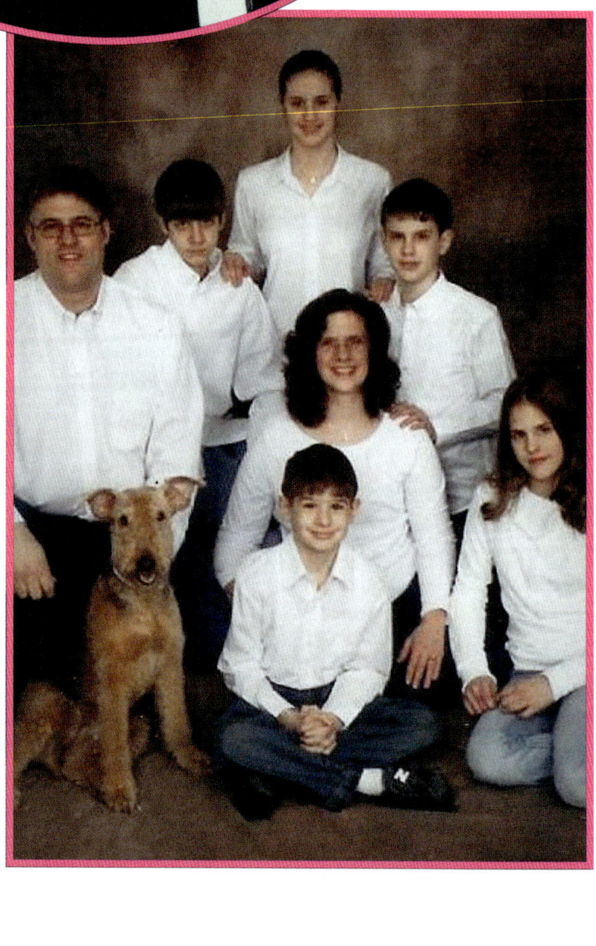

Mary Kowatch and her family. Photo by Expresions, Schofield, Wis

Gene and Karen Nelson on vacation in Jamaica soon after chemotherapy and radiation in 2005

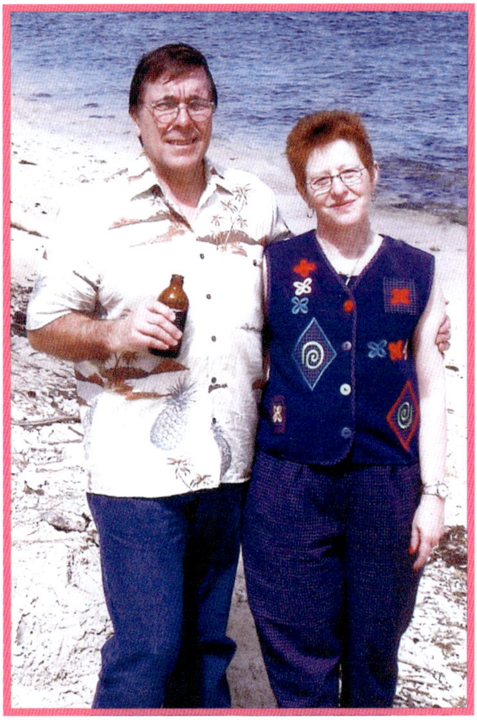

Mother's Day 2006 – Karen and her husband, Gene, with their grandchildren

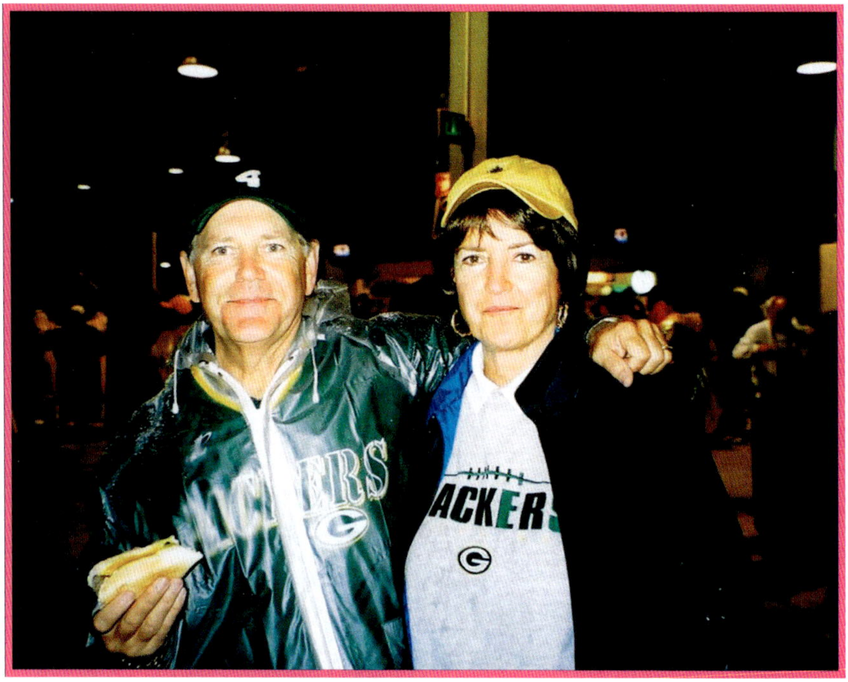

Beverly Testin and her husband, William, at a Green Bay Packer game.
Bev's comments, "No eyebrows, painted brows and a wig!"

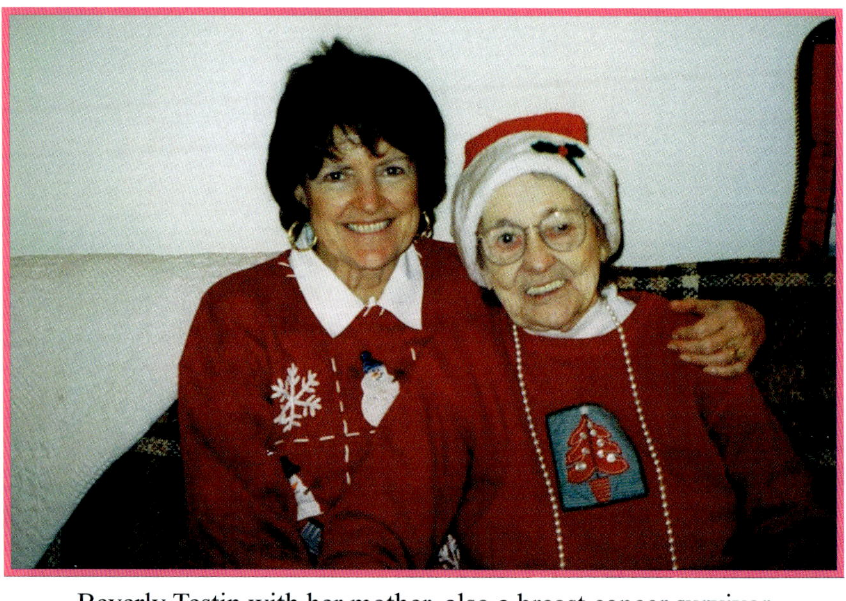

Beverly Testin with her mother, also a breast cancer survivor

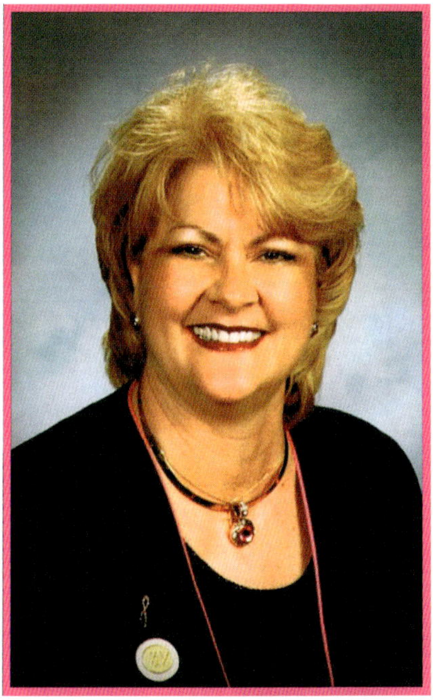

Diane Plantenberg

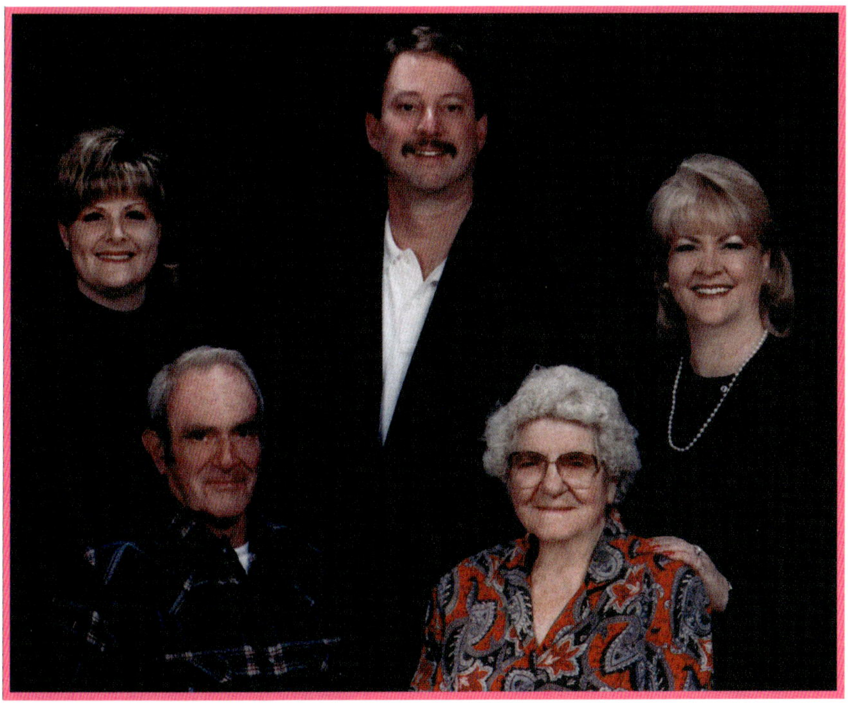

Diane Plantenberg and family, Tracy, Dennis, Diane, Duane and Grandma Irma

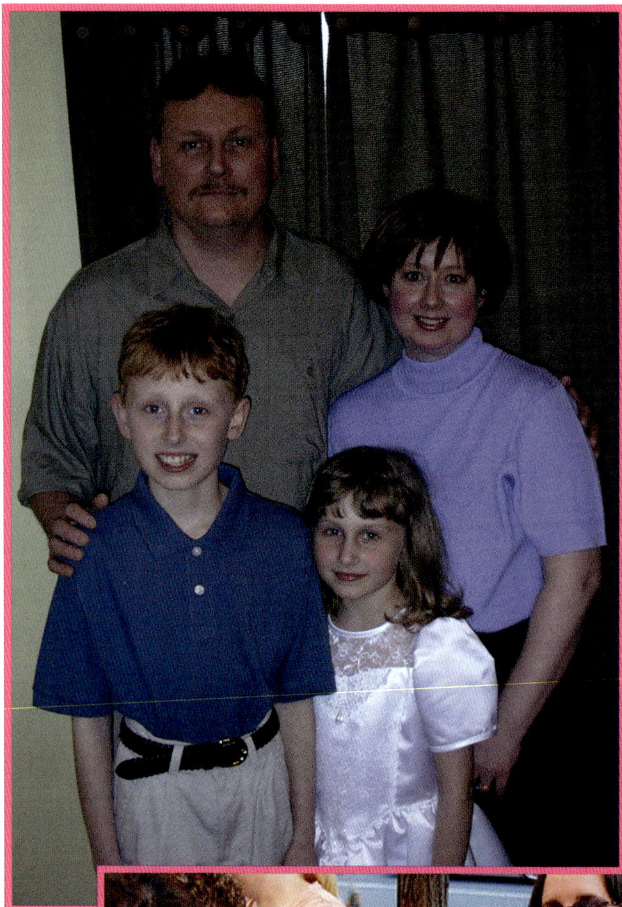

Amy White and her family — husband, Scott, and children, Daniel and Laurel

Amy and her mother, Rae Ellen Reekie, also a breast cancer survivor

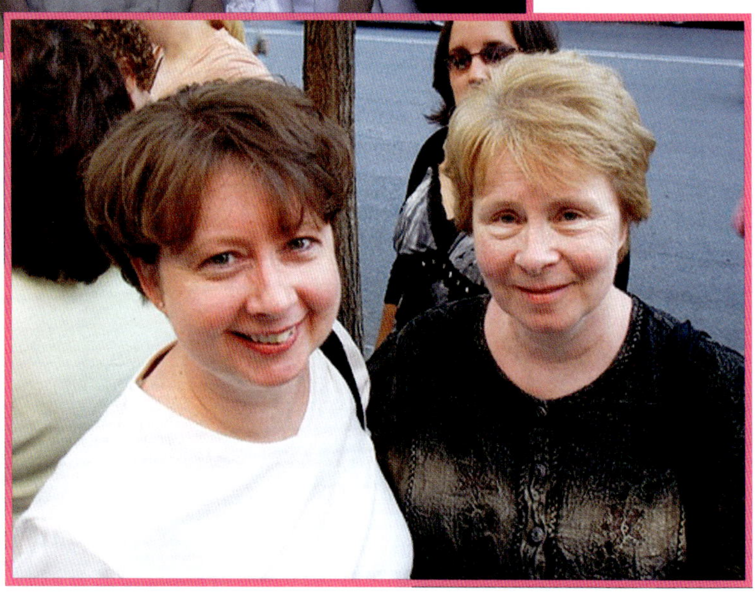

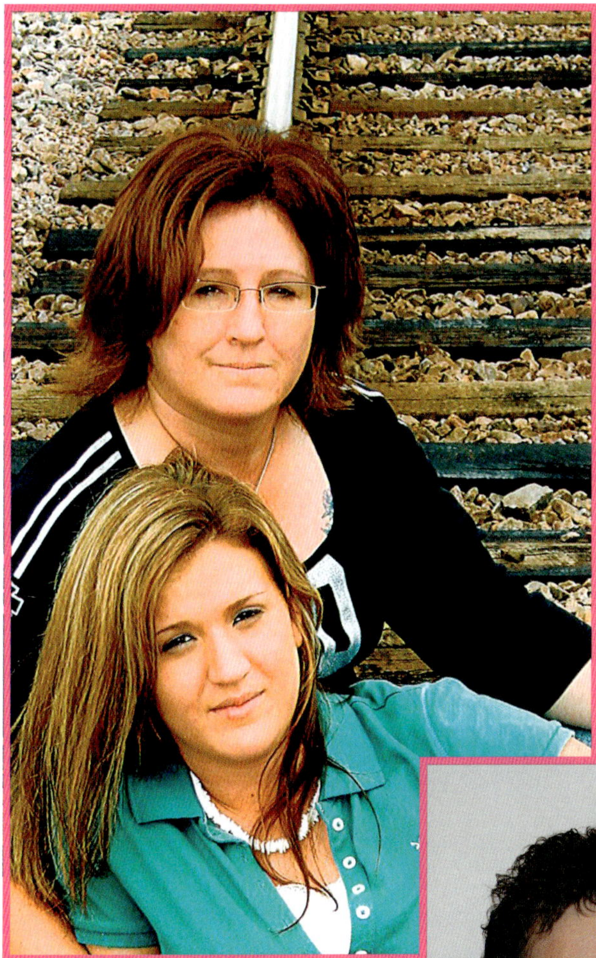

Rose Storkel and her daughter

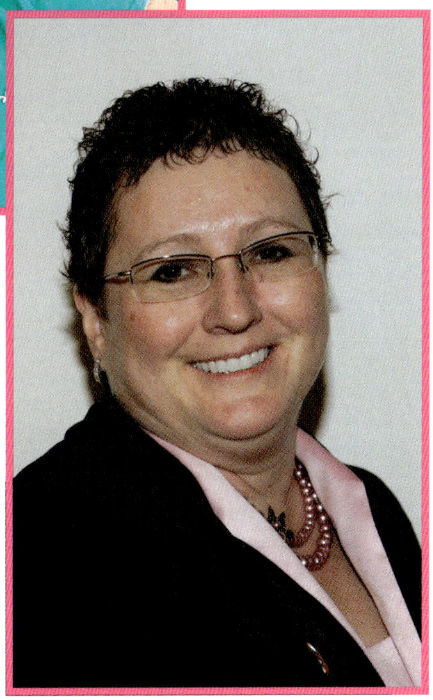

Rose Storkel at the LeRoy Butler Foundation Spring Fling, April 2007

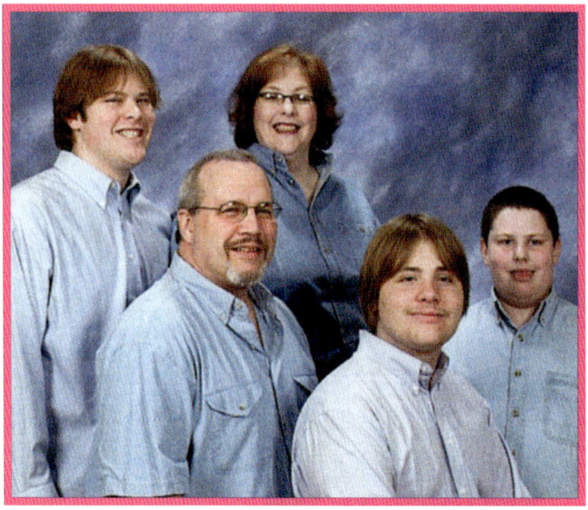

Heidi Schoenberger, her husband, Eric, and the boys

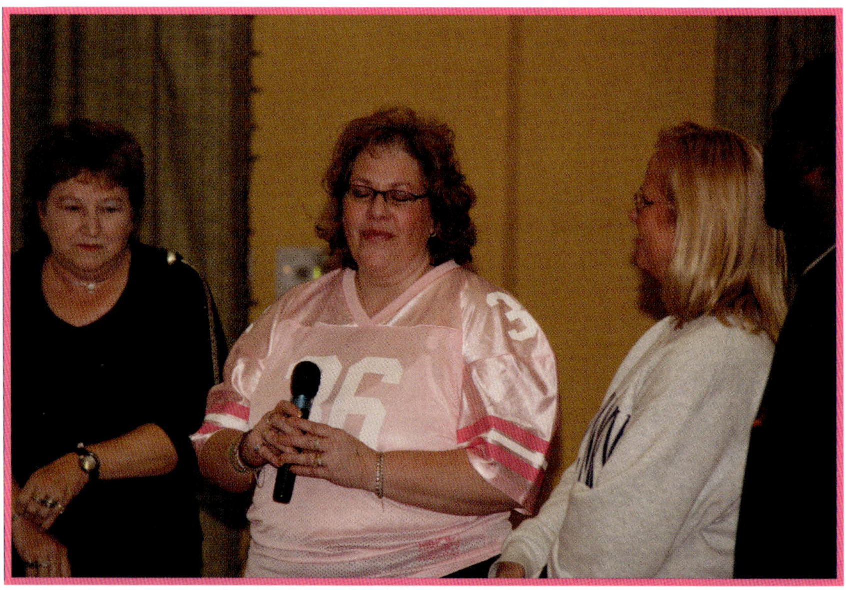

Heidi Schoenberger told her story at the "Battle of the Borders" event. It was an emotional time for all.

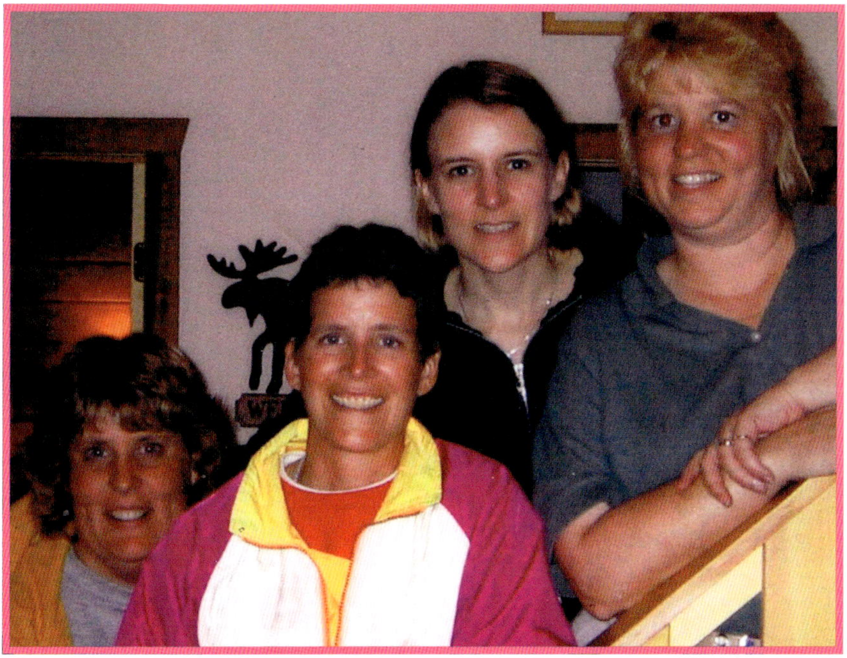

The circle of friends, from left,
Wanda, Shelly Duncan Bowman, Beth and Deneen

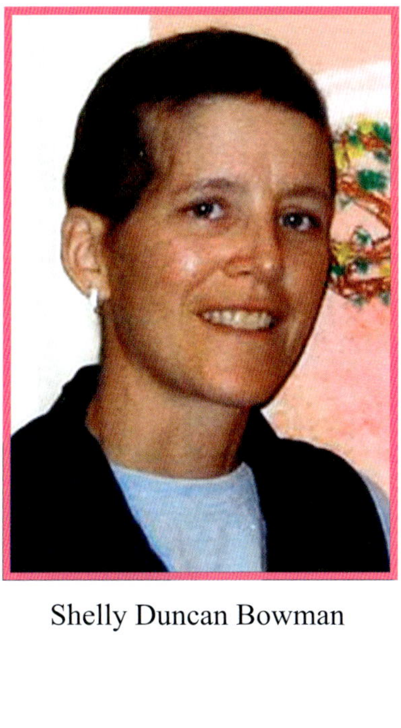

Shelly Duncan Bowman

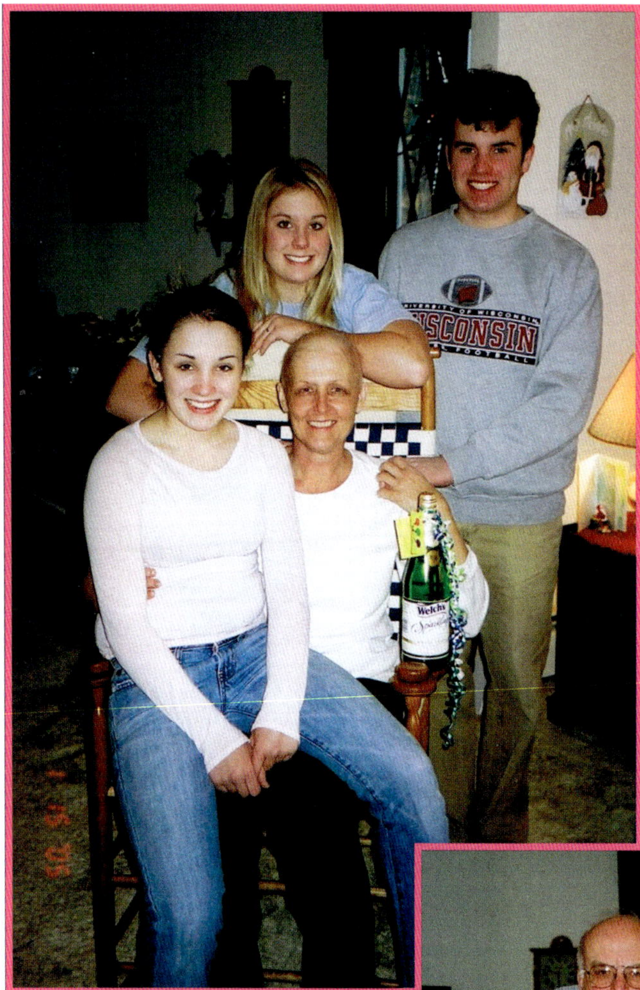

Jan. 15, 2005 — the last of the 16-week chemotherapy treatments. Anne Jacobson celebrates with her three children, Paul, Leslie and Catherine

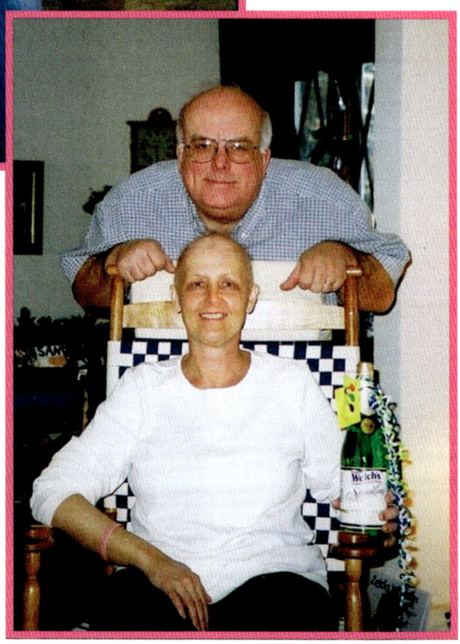

Anne with her devoted husband, LaMont

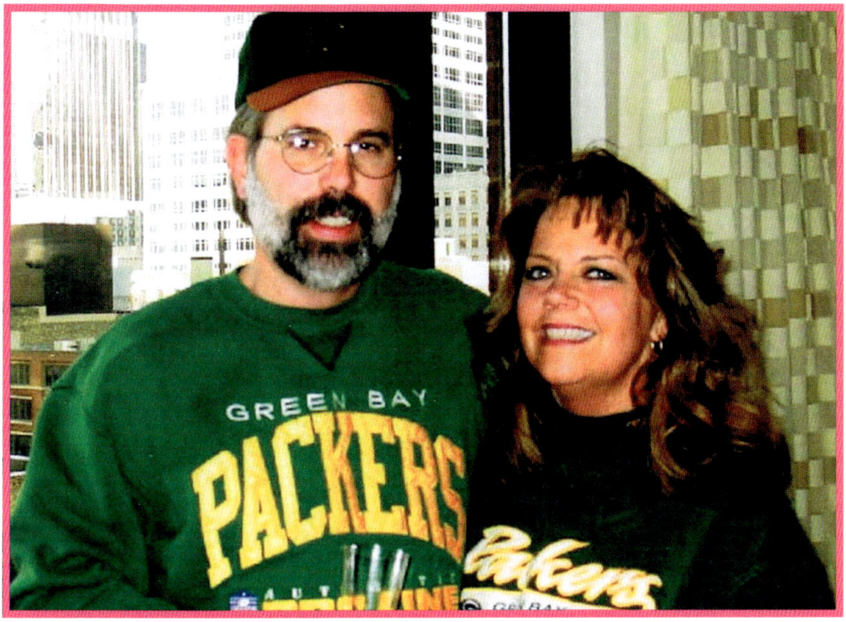

Sondra Clinkscales and her husband Rick, both Green Bay Packer fans

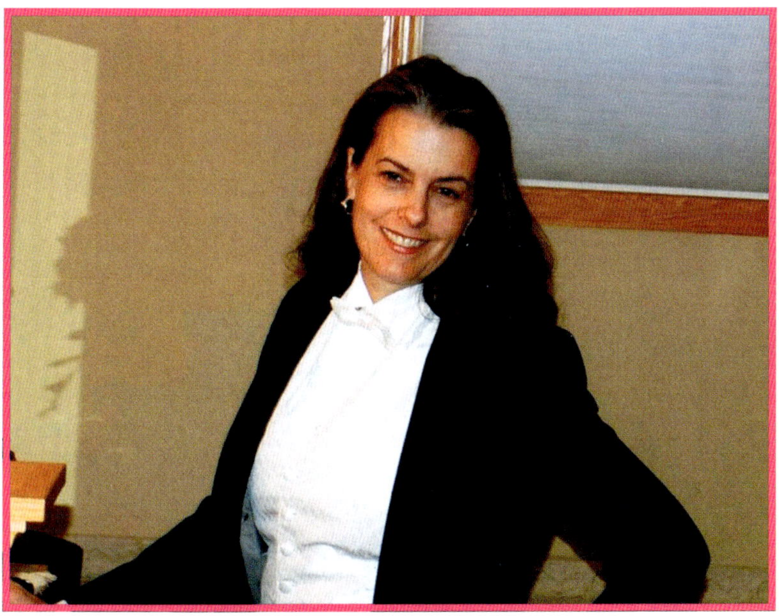

Christine Kennelly, Sondra's sister

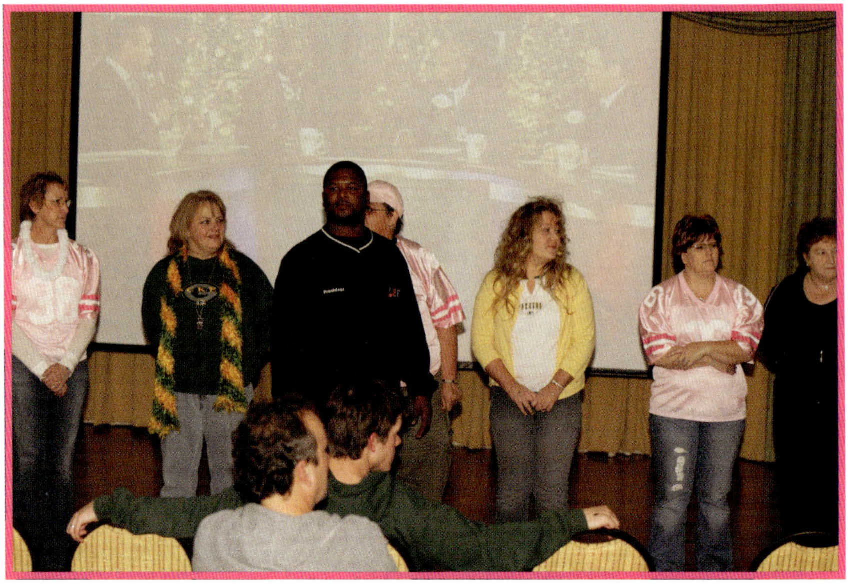

LeRoy Butler was host of the "Battle of the Borders" event in Warrens, Wis., December 2006. Photos by Bonnie Wood

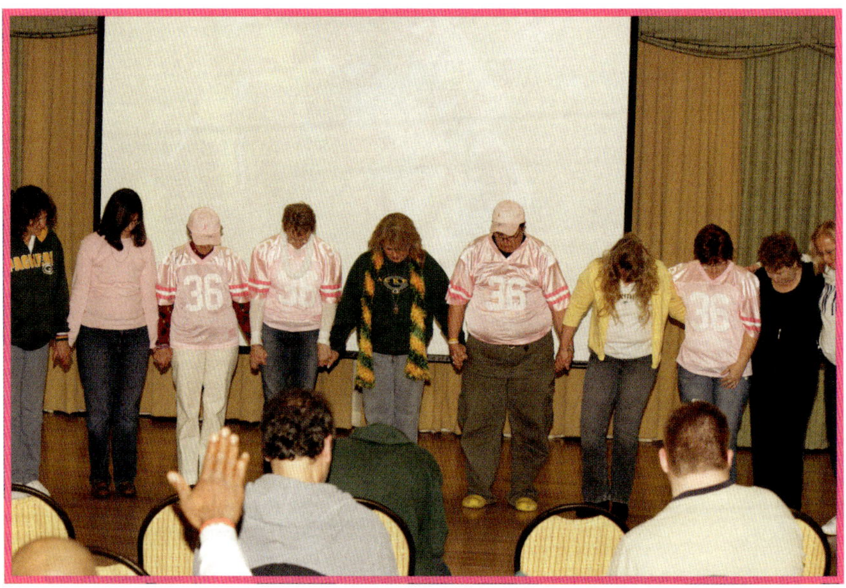

Many of the women featured in this book were in attendance at the December 2006 event. They shared their stories of hope and courage.

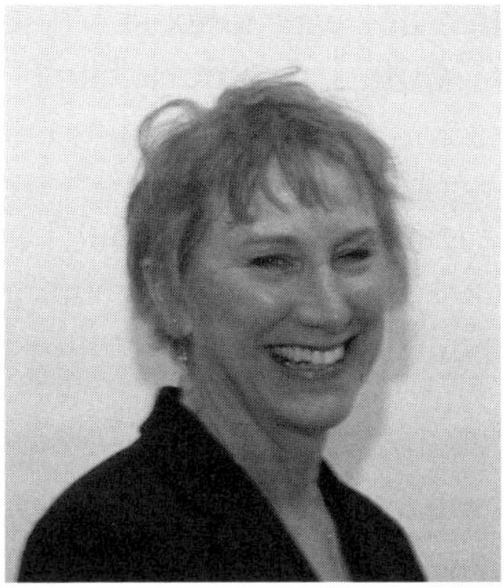

Chapter Seven

The Realities of Cancer

By Ursula Koxlien, Galesville, Wis.

Life was pretty normal for me in 2004. I was your average middle-aged woman in Middle America. My family is the usual variety of the American family with a loving husband and two wonderful children. We live in an idyllic country setting outside of a small Midwestern town. We were all happy with our normally pleasant lives. Little did we know that our pleasant lives were soon to become unpleasantly disrupted…

The first sign of trouble came in early spring. It showed as an exaggerated version of that tenderness one can get in the breasts. I just figured it was due to menopausal hormonal changes. I didn't worry because I had always heard that "cancer doesn't hurt." But by the first part of May, the pain didn't go away and a hard swelling was developing. Now I was worried. I called my physician immediately. She referred me to a breast cancer specialist who referred me immediately to the cancer center.

I went through the usual tests. The mammogram was excruciatingly painful but showed nothing. Then came an ultrasound, and finally three biopsies. It took the biopsies to confirm that I had cancer. There was almost a sense of relief to finally find out the diagnosis. Living with uncertainty while waiting for results of the tests was a dreadful way to exist. At least now I could move on to what was next. Still, I was devastated. My lovely normal life was falling apart.

The whirlwind of tests, and finding out I had cancer was just the beginning. There was so much more to comprehend -- the details of my type of cancer and the treatment options. My cancer -- a large mass, stage three and very invasive -- indicated what type of treatment would be best for my situation. The options were having a mastectomy or lumpectomy, followed by chemotherapy and radiation. I could have just the surgery and see what happened, then do chemo and radiation later. Or, I could start with chemo and radiation, waiting to see if I needed surgery later. All options came with a different percentage of survival. I had the best chance for survival if I did the most aggressive treatment.

It was all so frightening and overwhelming. I was in shock and often in a daze. I kept hoping that it was all just a dream and that I would wake up and be back in my normal, happy life. I was hearing what all the doctors were saying, but I had a hard time processing all the medical talk. My husband translated for me. He was right there helping me through all the tests and discussions. He was jovial in translating the information, but behind the facade, I could see he was as afraid as I was. His normal little world was falling apart also.

I spent lots of time sobbing after doctor visits. I was incessantly troubled about what options to take. The length of the treatment depended on what option I chose. It was mind-boggling. We needed some help. Since I was so confident in my surgeon, I asked her what she would do. She leveled with me and said that she would go with the most aggressive option: surgery, chemo, and radiation. She said that she would not want regrets; she would want to see her kids grow up. Even though the most aggressive is the toughest treatment and makes you the sickest, it is the most thorough and gives the best chances for survival. Finally reality was setting in. I was making the most important choices of my life. We chose to go with the most aggressive approach.

It was time now to tell our children the news. My son was a freshman in college, home on summer break. My daughter was in her last days as a freshman in high school. They knew of the trips to the doctor but had no idea what was going on. It fell to me to tell them. My husband couldn't find the words.

It is a very awful situation to have to tell your kids. Finding the words was so overwhelming that I found myself crying before I could even speak. So there I sat, sobbing. They were shocked to see their mother crying. I could see the fear and anxiety in their faces. Finally, the story all came out -- the diagnosis and what was to come. We all cried and hugged. They needed reassurance that I wasn't going to die today. Life would continue, however, not in the normal, pleasant life we were accustom to. They needed to know that their love and support would be crucial in my recovery. In the coming months, they really stepped up to the task. Many times their young, optimistic view of the world was uplifting and proved to be very important in my treatment and recovery.

Now for the hardest part. My surgery was done the first part of June. I had a radical mastectomy of the right breast and sixteen lymph nodes removed. Four of the nodes proved to be cancerous. While they were at it, they did the initial stage for reconstruction. Luckily, on waking up, I didn't have to feel any pain because I had an epidural block. I was feeling no pain from the shoulders down. The first thing I remember on waking was the looks on the faces of my husband and children, disbelief and worry. Although we tried to prepare the children for the trauma of post-surgery, the reality of seeing their mother hooked up to tubes; looking battered and in and out of consciousness filled them with fear.

During my six day post surgical recovery in the hospital, I didn't lack for love from family and friends. My room was filled with the flowers of June from friends' gardens as well as the encouraging faces of visitors. This really helped keep my spirits up as I was gradually brought out of the pain mediation. The hospital staff was wonderful, being very attentive and encouraging.

The treatment phase began six weeks later. All together the chemo lasted 19 weeks, with an additional 33 days of radiation.

Some weeks I was too sick to have a chemo treatment. The first set of drugs gave me a severe allergic reaction. I was extremely nauseous, accompanied by an overwhelming need to rest. My doctor immediately put me on a drug for nausea. But by the second chemotherapy treatment, they had figured out how to keep me from being so sick. Pre-chemo I was given an IV of anti-allergen drugs, followed by a saline flush. I felt like a walking pharmacy with all the drugs I was using --drugs for nausea, for sore bones, for another allergic reaction on my skin, and drugs for keeping all the drugs down. The toll on my body was devastating.

By the first week of August, my hair was falling out. My son and I had a pact that we would shave our heads together once that started. First, I shaved his head, then he shaved mine -- but only if I wouldn't cry. He said, "If you cry, I won't shave your head." We picked out our "do" rags. He had a ZZ Top bandana. Mine was pink and scratchy. We then went on vacation up to a cabin on a Wisconsin lake. I took along an assortment of hats to continue a lighthearted attitude about losing my hair. When I returned to work I used wigs fitted and styled by a woman who worked with cancer patients. I had a very public job as a front desk office manager and I didn't want people to be asking why I was wearing a "do" rag.

During this whole treatment time, I felt like I was living my life in a fog. I remember one day lying in my bed, with the warm fall sunshine filtering through the drapes, completely exhausted from the most recent treatment. I would drift in and out of sleep in a semi-conscious state. My daughter very quietly tiptoed into the bedroom to check on me. She lowered her head towards my chest to listen for the sound of my breathing. I could smell the fresh scent of sunshine on her hair as it brushed gently across by face. I knew she was there, but I was unable to respond to tell her that I was OK.

She must have been concerned that I wasn't breathing, because soon after she left, my husband came slowly creeping into the bedroom. I could hear the heavier footsteps as he came to my side of the bed. Then I felt the light touch of his hand on my chest. Again, I was unable to respond and soon all was quiet.

On Dec. 31, I had my last radiation treatment. The year from hell was over! I had done every thing I could to survive. Now I could try to resume a "normal" life. It was a good way to start a new year. It was time to begin working on getting healthy again. I began paying attention to getting proper nutrition and started an exercise program. It was important to begin slowly with exercise since I was so weak from all the treatment. My goal for that year was to get healthy enough to undergo the second phase and completion of reconstruction. I wanted to have a feeling of being whole again. I was glad to get back to my normally pleasant life with my family and idyllic country home without the daily disruptions of the active cancer treatment.

It has now been three years since the trouble began. So far, my body shows no signs of harboring the disease. I continue to try to live a healthy, relaxed lifestyle. My odyssey is a reality I will always live with. As is often told, this life threatening experience helped me to appreciate all the treasures of my life -- my family and friends, the nature around me. I want to live each day in the present and to the absolute fullest, to make decisions without regrets, to be honest about my feelings and let people know how I feel about them, to not wait for a special occasion to use the good china, to live every day as if it is the most important day of my life.

Reflections from a cancer survivor's daughter
By Ursula Koxlien's daughter

I have had to live this past year in a mind set not my own. One I wouldn't wish on my worst enemy. What in this world and beyond could cause that? An evil six-letter word that strikes even the strongest -- CANCER. My one phrase of advice about cancer -- don't act like you know or think how it affects other people; you won't and never will, unless it gets your mother, father, sister, brother or immediate family. It's something you have to experience to understand, you can't read a book or watch a movie and know how to handle it.

As I said before, last year I was not myself. Just ask any of my friends who really paid attention to me. At the end of the school year I had to tell myself when I woke up that I needed to get though the day with a smile on my face no matter what happened. I hated leaving home and I hated coming back to it. I hated listening to girls talk about how much they hated their parents for not letting them go out last weekend. I hated listening to girls complaining about how horrible their mom's were. I hated the whole year from May 29th on.

On May 29th my mom, the woman who never got sick because she was too strong, sat us down after dinner, broke in to tears and told us the worst new that ever came out of her mouth, "I have breast cancer." I knew it wasn't good news before she even said it. I had never seen my mom cry before that. Once she said those words, I broke into tears. She told us all about how, and she told us what she knew about it. She told us that if we stayed strong we would get through this together. We knew that she was telling herself that more than she was telling us that. Within a few days, we had papers all over our table. On these papers were the percent chances of survival with each method used. None of them were over 55 percent chance of survival after 10 years. To me, I thought I was going to lose my mom before I got married. I couldn't help but think that she wouldn't sit in a pew at my wedding and cry her eyes out (tears of joy of course) or that she wouldn't be here to see my first child. I wanted her to be the one that didn't fit with the stats. I wanted and needed her to stick around for a long time, because I knew that I would need her help and guidance and her presence. I knew that if she didn't make it though this I would become a complete wreck.

I had to keep going to school. That was one of the worst parts about it. I was really quiet and I avoided my friends because I didn't want their pity, what good would it do me? It wouldn't make things better; it wouldn't make it all go away like a bad dream. It would just make them feel weird around me and I didn't need that. I needed to just be normal, or as normal as I could be. I needed my friend to stay normal around me. I needed them so bad it hurt sometimes. I wanted to shout it out at the top of my lungs. I needed a way to get it off my shoulders. I had to stay focused during class, so that helped me take my mind off of the facts of my life. But as soon as the bell rang after 90 minutes of focusing on things other that this horrible fact, it all came flooding back into my mind.

Lunch was the worst time of my day. A week after we got our news, I was sitting at a table in our gym and I broke down into tears. I couldn't tell people why I was crying. I just shrugged it off and said that I just needed to have a cry. I couldn't hide that fact that something was wrong from my friends. My mom told me that if I really needed to talk to someone to go to the guidance office and talk to them about it. What good was that going to do? I knew that if I went in that office the entire high school staff would find out, and then the entire student body would know about it. I decided that I would keep it all in and I would find my own ways to deal with it. Why would I want to talk to someone who has no idea about how I feel? I thought I could just hold it all in until I was ready to deal with it. I didn't think that doing that would change me. Was I wrong -- that's when I got quiet and didn't want to live my real life anymore.

On June 4th, Mom had her first surgery. I thought that when we went to visit her it would be like it was on TV shows, but to my rude awaking it was nothing like it. I walked into that room and saw my mom hooked up to machines to make sure she was breathing and that her heart kept beating. She has four or five IV's hooked up to her arms and some weird compression things hooked up to both her legs. She wasn't awake yet from the surgery.

I just stood there dead silent. I thought that if I said anything something bad would happen. Tears started to roll down my cheeks and my brother put his arms around me. After what seems to be hours she woke up. My dad was sitting next to her bed in the chair. Mom looked at him motioned for a metal container and puked in it. I couldn't believe that my mom was sick in the hospital and puking, and there was nothing that I could do to help her. All I could do was watch as my dad held the metal pan for her. The entire time we were at the hospital my mom would wake up, puke and then go back to sleep. Every now and then a nurse would come in and check her drip bags and her vitals.

Reluctantly at 7 p.m. my dad took my brother and I home and we had to leave Mom there.

That was the first time I had ever left my Mom anywhere.

Features of hereditary breast cancer include:

- *Premenopausal breast cancer*
- *Two or more close relatives affected with breast or ovarian cancer at any age*
- *Multiple cancers (i.e. breast and ovarian cancer)*
- *Bilateral breast cancer*
- *Male breast cancer*

Everyone has BRCA1 and BRCA2 genes. When these genes are working, they prevent tumors from forming. Mutations in the genes are what predispose us to both breast and ovarian cancer. BRCA1 and BRCA2 are two of the 30,000 genes that we have in every cell of our body.

- *Christina Zaleski, MS, CGC, Senior Genetic Counselor, Marshfield Clinic, Wis.*

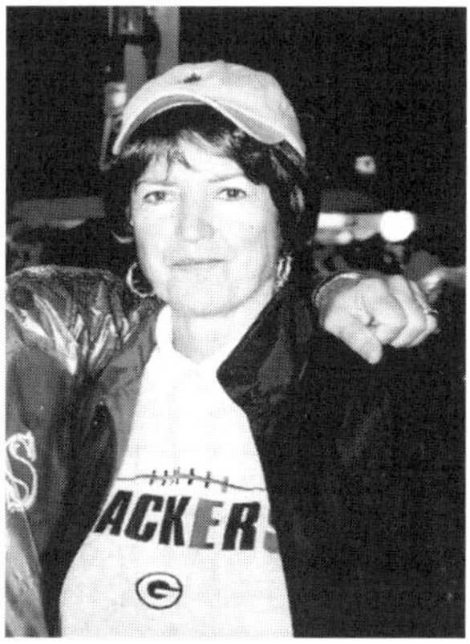

Chapter Eight

Prepared For A Challenge

By Beverly Testin, Manitowish Waters, Wis.

When I heard the words breast cancer, I was recuperating from Acoustic Neuroma brain tumor surgery. This is a very rare brain tumor that affects all your facial nerves, hearing, swallowing, taste and balance. After an eight and one-half hour surgery, I was told the tumor was not malignant; my balance nerve had been removed and I had at least 75 percent hearing loss in my left ear. The loud buzzing tinnitus would be there forever, and my complete recovery would take up to two years. As I think back, this serious brain tumor experience prepared me for what was to come next.

In October of 2002, I found a large mass on my left breast. At that time I was part of the Star study at the Marshfield Clinic in Marshfield, Wis. This study was for women who were at very high risk for breast cancer. The fact that I had never had children, plus my mother having breast cancer, made me a candidate for the study. I joined and received one extra office call and breast exam by a surgeon every year paid for by the study.

I drove 250 miles and got in to see the doctor the same day I found the lump. I was given a breast exam and also a mammogram and told it was nothing. Two months later I had my annual physical and after examining my breast, the doctor had a very worried look on his face. He said there was definitely something there and that I needed to see the surgeon, who was also the Star study surgeon. This time I had an ultrasound, a needle biopsy and an exam by the surgeon. I remember raising my arms and showing him that my breasts seemed asymmetrical. One breast was rounded at the bottom and the other was flat. He didn't seem to notice. He told me the ultrasound showed nothing, and it felt like normal breast tissue. His office called several days later to tell me the needle biopsy was fine and I should return in six months.

During those months I had little time to think about myself. My dad had a heart attack, and at age 87, underwent heart surgery. He had four bypasses and a new heart valve. My dad was the sole caregiver for my mother, who had dementia. We ended up putting her in an assisted living while my dad resided in the physical therapy unit of Wausau Hospital. My dad passed away shortly after and my mother was placed in a nursing home.

Years earlier my mother had been diagnosed with breast cancer at the age of 85. When I had found out that she was due for her annual physical, I asked my dad if Mother had ever had a mammogram. His answer was, "I don't think so." We got it scheduled and both my dad and I went along. I will never forget that day. After the mammogram they asked us to stop at the front desk. They handed me a card and said, "Your mother has one more appointment." I looked at the doctor's name and saw he was a surgeon. That could only mean one thing. My heart began to race and I tried to hold back the tears. I was in the room when the doctor showed us the x-ray with the tumor and said, "Your mother has breast cancer." He knew this without doing a biopsy.

We all cried. My immediate thought was she was going to die. I also remember thinking that now I was also at high risk. The next week my mother underwent a lumpectomy and also had her lymph nodes removed. After her surgery I stayed with my folks. I knew my dad would not be able to handle the situation. I drained and measured her tubes, changed her bandages, etc. All the same things my husband ended up doing for me. Because the nodes were clear, she would not have chemotherapy, just five weeks of radiation. Mother did not tolerate the radiation very well. It made her tired and dizzy, but she got through it. I remember when she hit the five year survivor mark. Without that mammogram she would not have celebrated her 99th birthday on Jan. 15, 2007.

I returned for my scheduled appointment in June of 2003. This time it was instantly obvious that something was wrong. The doctor sent me for a needle biopsy to be done with the aid of an ultrasound to make sure they didn't miss the area in question. The doctor called me the next day and said all four samples taken from different areas of my breast were malignant. I needed a bone scan at once to see if it had spread. Once again I drove 250 miles roundtrip to Marshfield, Wis., had my scan and saw the doctor. My bones looked clear, but they couldn't be 100 percent sure because they had nothing to compare it to.

I was told I would need surgery, chemotherapy and possibly radiation. I never cried, but I was scared and angry. How could this have been missed? Eight months had passed since I first found the lump in my breast. I knew I had to deal with this at once. I had been there before with the brain tumor and I would remain strong and keep a positive attitude. I was not going to die of breast cancer.

I decided to get a second opinion. In this process my x-rays were lost and this whole fiasco cost me about two weeks. The diagnosis was the same and I was set up for surgery and reconstruction the end of July. As the days passed, I was an emotional wreck. All I could think about was the fact that I have cancer. Why am I waiting seven weeks? The surgeon could get me in, but the plastic surgeon was booked solid. Both doctors often worked together and didn't seem to think there was a need to rush. I finally took the matter into my own hands, called a retired doctor friend and asked his opinion. He gave me the name of a surgeon in Wausau, Wis. I called and saw her at 6 p.m. the next evening after she had finished with all of her other patients. She explained everything to me in detail and suggested I get the surgery as soon as possible. Since the cancer was so widespread in my breast, she told me she would be removing all my lymph nodes.

This was a Thursday and she did the surgery on the following Tuesday, four weeks after my diagnosis. I was hospitalized overnight and sent home the next day with four drain tubes and lots of bandages. My husband was my nurse for the next two weeks. He measured and emptied all my drain tubes twice daily. Several days later I received a call from my surgeon telling me the cancer had spread to the lymph nodes and I would have to see an oncologist for further treatment. Because one of the malignant areas was very close to my chest wall, she was also going to recommend radiation therapy after I completed the chemotherapy.

I saw the oncologist three weeks after my surgery. He began by telling me that my cancer was lobular and contained the overactive gene called HER2. Only 25 percent of the breast cancers are of this more aggressive type. Next he gave me my statistics. I thought I was hearing things when he told me that without further treatment there was a 60 percent chance that the cancer would return somewhere in my body within five years, and probably sooner. He urged me to join a random study that would include the usual six months of chemotherapy, plus one year of a drug called Herceptin. After reading the two pages of side effects of the chemotherapy, I now had another page of the side effects from the Herceptin. I decided to join the study, but prayed that I would not be chosen for the Herceptin. Only my oncologist was disappointed when I wasn't chosen. Even though I didn't receive the drug, I would still have to have a periodic MUGA scan to check the heart for possible side effects. The study paid for all the extras and my insurance covered the chemotherapy. I paid for my insurance and my deductible.

The following week I entered the hospital for day surgery to have a port placed so I could begin receiving chemotherapy the next day. I remember walking into the chemotherapy room as frightened as I had ever been in my life. My chemotherapy was scheduled every three weeks for six months. It would take five to six hours. On occasion my mother-in-law would be in the chair next to me, also receiving treatment for breast cancer. My husband was always there for both of us. I really can't say enough about my husband. He has driven me to every doctor's appointment, 28 radiation treatments and 56 chemo treatments. He has also been dealing with his mother's breast cancer for the past five years.

I had been told my hair would begin to fall out the third week. Well on the tenth day my hair was falling out in chunks. I lived in a small town and had to travel a distance to the nearest salon that sold wigs. This salon had a huge ad in the phone book, so I knew I would be able to find something. Turns out they had one wig in my size for $385. Even though I hated the wig, I took it because I knew my hair would be gone in a few days. The salon took advantage of me because of my desperate situation. The University of Wisconsin Cancer Center in Madison, Wis. no longer lists this salon. The American Cancer Society has a booklet, which I would highly recommend, with reasonably priced wigs. The Look Good Feel Better program is wonderful for those going through chemotherapy.

My side effects, besides hair loss, included mouth sores, numbness and tingling in my feet, mood swings, difficulty sleeping and on several occasions, a mild nausea feeling. I continued my normal daily activities, including exercise. The third day was always my tired day. The rest of the time I was ready to go. People I barely knew were stopping me on the street, calling, sending cards, books, etc. I finished my last chemotherapy two days before Christmas and the following week had my port removed. That was the best present I could have had.

My next appointment would be in two weeks, January 2004, with the radiologist. The first appointment was the planning visit. A special machine called a simulator mapped out my treatment plan. Tiny permanent tattoos were marked on my chest so that the radiation beam would be in the exact same place every time. I was scheduled for five weeks of radiation every day except weekends. I traveled 170 miles roundtrip. When the weather was bad we would stay overnight. A side effect from the radiation was lymphedema during the last week of treatment. This is a swelling of the arm on the affected side and requires physical therapy. I still have flair ups, and battle the insurance to pay. It seems the more qualified the technician, the less likely the insurance will pay. I was just recently stuck with a $1,000 bill, which the insurance refused to cover.

Since my mother had breast cancer, my oncologist sent me to the University of Wisconsin Clinical Genetics Center for a conference. I had to gather information on my mother's eight sisters, six brothers and numerous cousins. This was not an easy task and involved many phone calls and explanations as to why I needed this information. To get a complete medical record the family has to fill out the request. After looking over my family history, they concluded that it was unlikely that my breast cancer was caused by a BRCA1 or BRCA2 breast cancer susceptibility mutation. Rather it appeared that the cancers in my family arose by chance, or were influenced by a combination of unknown environmental and/or low-risk genetic factors.

In April of 2005, the data from the Herceptin study was made available to the public. The studies showed that Herceptin improved the chance of being alive and free of cancer by 52 percent when given in conjunction with chemotherapy. Shortly after the news broke, I received a letter from the study informing me that the study would pay for Herceptin for anyone that was no more than six months out from chemotherapy. That excluded me because I had finished my chemotherapy 14 months ago. My doctor wanted me to proceed with the Herceptin. My husband and I discussed it. Another port, another year of weekly treatments, weekly blood work and weekly doctor's appointments and more MUGA scans. The cost would be close to $100,000, not including my weekly travel time and gas. What if the insurance wouldn't pay? My doctor made the call and somehow persuaded the insurance company to pay. I immediately had my port put back in and began my treatments. I finished in May of 2006. This was three years after my initial diagnosis.

In September of 2002, just one month before I first discovered the lump on my breast, my husband received a call that his 89-year old mother had taken a fall and was in the emergency room about 175 miles away. The emergency room doctor called to let us know that nothing was broken, but he suggested she see an oncologist as soon as possible because he was certain she had breast cancer. We were both in a total state of shock.

We immediately drove to see her and got her in to see a doctor. The diagnosis was confirmed – she had breast cancer and it had spread to her bones. At the time she lived alone in a small town and was no longer driving. We paid the neighbor to care for her so she could remain in her own home. The decisions we had to make were not easy. We felt she needed to be closer to us, so we ended up moving her into an assisted living right near the Wausau Hospital.

Because of her age, the oncologist, who also turned out to be my doctor, decided against surgery. He kept her alive the last four years with oral cancer medications and IV injections every three weeks to strengthen her bones. She had a very good quality of life until December of 2006 when her condition began to deteriorate. We were forced to move her to the nursing home. The oncologist gave her a few months. It was tough watching her grow weaker and get more confused day by day. She was no longer eating and slept most of the time. On Jan. 29, 2007, my mother-in-law, Honor Testin Brown, passed away from mestastic breast cancer.

When I heard the word breast cancer, I knew I was in for a long haul. I never dreamed the expenses that would be involved. The total for all my treatments, surgery, scans, doctors, meds, travel time and gas was almost $200,000. In June of 2007, it will be four years. I still see my surgeon and oncologist for blood work, exams and scans every three months. My out of pocket expenses have been huge, but fortunately I have been able to handle them. I think often about those with little or no insurance and the decisions they are forced to make.

Going from brain tumor to breast cancer and dealing with all the issues involved has had a great impact on my perspective of life. I understand how important it is to have faith in God and support of your family and friends. Beating this terrible disease is not an easy task. I endured a lot of pain, both physically and emotionally, but through it all I remained positive.

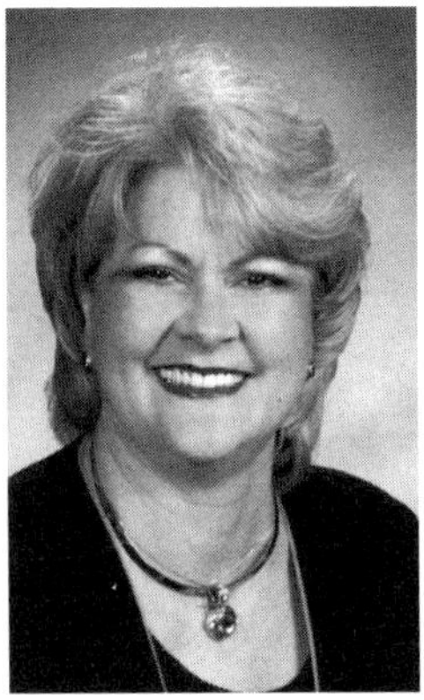

Chapter Nine

My Journey with the Big "C"

By Diane Plantenberg, Wonewoc, Wis.

In April 2003 I scheduled my yearly *routine* mammogram. I wanted to get in and get it done before I had to go into the fields to plant crops. We were doing pick your own strawberries and I had beef cattle at the time.

April 7, 2003 -- from that date on, nothing in my life would be *routine* again.

A week later I received a letter telling me something looked suspicious and they wanted me to return for more follow up x-rays. The x-rays were not conclusive, so I was scheduled for an MRI the following week. When the nurses came to get me to take me to the room where the MRI machine was, they said the machine would be loud. Well, you have to lay face down and put each breast in a hole. So OK, by now I am in hysterics – laughing. Being a farm girl, the machine sounded like a milking machine. The nurses got a kick out of that.

The MRI was also inconclusive, it showed something but they couldn't tell for sure. The next week I was scheduled for an ultrasound. When you look at the ultrasound screen, normal tumors show up a solid color, but when cancer is present, the tumor has a different color around it.

They asked me that day if I wanted to do the biopsy right then or come back? As you know, waiting to do these tests is very nerve-racking. I said, "Lets get it done, I'm here." Getting a biopsy is very painful, it took the doctor four tries to get enough tissue to feel comfortable, and comfort was not high on my list. Then they push on the area to make sure you don't get a hematoma -- that was fun. Well we were getting closer, now the waiting game for the results. By now it was the first week of May.

You try to tell yourself it will all be OK, but inside you're scared to death what the results will be -- and you don't want to scare yourself, so you keep busy doing anything you can until someone calls.

I had to wait until the Monday morning after Mother's Day; I will never forget answering the phone that morning and the doctor telling me, "It's positive, you have breast cancer."

My husband held me and we both cried.

It feels like someone just kicked you in the stomach. I was thinking, "No, not me." I was scared, but I didn't have time to think about it for long. They had already scheduled for me to meet with the surgeon, and my surgery date was already set. My surgeon was awesome; she explained everything I would go through in very plain language.

The following Wednesday, I did my prep. And on Thursday, I went for my nuclear test. They inject nuclear dye into the breast 24 hours before surgery. On the day of surgery, a blue dye is injected into the breast and that follows the nuclear dye, so the surgeon knows which lymph nodes to take first.

On Friday morning, May 30, 2003, I went for surgery. It was 6 a.m. and the nurses were prepping me. They thought I was crazy because I was giving our daughter paperwork and directions to finish my third month of DIQ in Mary Kay Cosmetics. DIQ is "director in qualifications." Everything had to be in that day, the last day of the month, and I was headed for surgery.

They take five lymph nodes at a time. If they are not clear, they take five more at a time until they get clear lymph nodes. I was lucky; my first five came out clear. My tumor was two and one-half centimeters in size. My tumor was also estrogen positive. I met with my oncologist, who by the way, travels all over the world teaching on breast cancer. He likes alternatives to chemotherapy, so he suggested I have a full hysterectomy, which would take all the estrogen out of my body, and leave nothing to feed any more tumors. Through his studies, he has found that when you have a hysterectomy mid-way through your cycle, the odds of cancer not reoccurring go from 80 percent to 93 percent.

In June I finished to be a Director with Mary Kay Cosmetics and in July I was scheduled to debut in Dallas, Texas on stage, which would be mid-cycle for me. So on August 15, 2003, I had a full hysterectomy, and would not have to go through chemotherapy -- Yeah!

The year 2003 was quite a roller coaster ride for me.

Since they cut me hip to hip for my hysterectomy, they called it the bikini cut. It was the third time I had been cut in the same spot. I had to wait eight weeks to heal before I started radiation treatments.

In October 2003, I went for my simulation session. These are tattoos for the radiology technicians to line up the machine just right and aim the beam where it needs to be without harming any internal organs.

On October 13, I started my treatments. Five days a week I drove to Madison, Wis., one and one-half hour one way for a 10-minute treatment. After four weeks I couldn't drive myself anymore. I have so many wonderful friends and family, they all pitched in and drove or rode with me. Even my then 102-year-old grandma went with me, and she likes to remind me we almost hit a deer in the middle of the day. You get very tired and your stomach gets queasy about an hour after each treatment. By the time you get to the last eight -- these are very intense -- your skin is red and burned from the radiation. The nurses I worked with are still great friends of mine to this day. They took the time to listen on the bad days and we laughed a lot on the good days. It's amazing what our bodies can endure and keep on ticking.

Now on an emotional level I really have to touch on my faith, and my Mary Kay training. God first, family second, career third. Once the shock was gone -- well not gone, but put aside -- I said a prayer to God to give me the strength I needed to get through this. My favorite quote is taken from Philippians, "I can do all things through Christ who strengthens me."

We all hope we will never have to go through the "Big C." I never had any doubt God would bring me through this adventure in my life. God delivers to us everything we need, whether it's on an emotional level, or a financial one.

It wasn't that easy for my family. My husband, Dennis, is one of the most loving and caring people I know, and I am truly lucky to be married to him. But this shook him to the core. Because he loves me so much, it was hard for him to watch me go through this and not be able to help me. It's hard because the people who love us want to fix everything for us, and this was out of his hands to fix. Feeling helpless is very hard. And the unknown of what the outcome of surgery would be is very scary. The fear that grips you is heart wrenching.

But I reassured him I wasn't leaving him soon. I just got him trained after 33 years of marriage. We have a timeless love. Family and faith go hand and hand!

We lost our home to fire in 1998. The fire marshal said we shouldn't have survived the fire, but God had bigger plans for us. And then five years later I was diagnosed with breast cancer. I am a three-year survivor, so once again God has plans for me. If I can help even one person get through their journey with breast cancer, I feel I have done what God intended me to do.

This also was hard for our daughter, Tracy. My mother died of cancer, multiple myeloma, at the age of 52. For those of you who don't know, multiple myeloma is not hereditary -- its common name is bone cancer. Tracy was very scared that she would lose me very young also. I was very sure I would be around for her wedding and her children -- to see her happy and successful. She is the light of my life.

Here are her feelings in her words: *"Well, where to begin. It started with a normal day at work, or what I thought was a normal day at work anyway. I was living about an hour away from my parents at the time and would go home about one or two times a week to see them. This particular day was one of my days to go home for a visit. Well, about half way through my day, my dad called to ask if I was coming home. I said yes, but didn't think too much of it because he does that a lot -- confirming with me, anyway.*

"Then about another hour later my Nana called to ask me the same thing. So at this point I was a little puzzled by the call, but dismissed it, thinking she wanted to see me about something as well, and I went about my day. Now mind you, my dad and Nana didn't tell me anything about what was going on, they just passed it off.

"Well, when my mom called a little later I knew something was up. So I started to question her, and this time I didn't let her off the hook. I finally got my answer, even though I wish I hadn't asked after I knew. She yelled at me, "Your mother has breast cancer." I felt like I had a ton of bricks dropped on me. I was waitressing at a restaurant in the Dells, and I will never forget where I was and what I was wearing, and what I was doing at that point. From that moment on, I was in a fog. I finally made it home a few hours later and life was never the same again.

"If I can get anything across to people who have this diagnosis, please share it with your family right away. My parents thought they were protecting me by not telling me right from the beginning, but in the long run it made it harder to deal with. I know they were trying to protect me, but it's easier to know from the beginning."

After I finished my treatments on January 8, 2004, the doctors told me everything looked good. The next day we took my dad in and were told he had pancreatic cancer. OK, now I fell apart. I was tired from my treatments and I couldn't fix this for my dad, who I have cared for since my mom died. My dad had a surgical procedure they called a "whipple." I truly believe in miracles now because he didn't do any treatments, and they gave him two years maximum. It was three years on February 3, 2007 and he is still with us. All his tests are still coming out good. He is diabetic now, but it is a small price to pay for having him with us. My father-in-law is also a cancer survivor, he had prostate cancer. And he is doing well.

Now another miracle is my grandmother. She turned 106 in May 2007, and she still lives on her farm, builds a wood fire in her stove every morning and gardens in the summer. Grams is a survivor. She had surgery on one breast in 1936, and in 1937 had surgery on the other breast. I truly believe grandma's secret is her outlook on life, she worries, but she also giggles a lot. She is my dad's mom. We have six generations. So now you can guess where a lot of my strength comes from. God has blessed us in so many ways. So is it any wonder I have a strong faith? And I got my grandma's personality in laughing a lot.

It's April 2004 and my scar is hurting a lot from the hysterectomy -- come to find out I have a hernia. The wall was weakened from surgery. So in September 2004, back to surgery I went for repair. It took a good six months to heal from this one. I wouldn't want to repeat that anytime soon.

Since I had a lot of time to read now, while recovering from surgery, I found a book that helped me a lot. *Just Get Me Through This!: The Practical Guide to Breast Cancer* by Deborah A. Cohen M.D., and Robert M. Gelfand. It's nice to read a book without all those big medical words we can't understand. After cancer you realize that the things that were important before are very trivial after. Our priorities are different. We realize what we could have lost, and were given a second chance to get it right. I have to express that when people found out I had breast cancer, the cards and flowers were overwhelming. I never realized how many lives I touched and how many people cared about me.

We make the time to smell the roses now!

What we give comes back to us ten-fold. And now I work to raise money for breast and other cancers. Helping and reassuring even one person on this journey is what it's all about.

God's blessings to everyone who reads this!

Family history is the most important way to determine if you are at risk for hereditary breast cancer. Breast and/or ovarian cancer on your father's side of the family is just as important as the same history on your mothers side of the family.

- Christina Zaleski, MS, CGC, Senior Genetic Counselor,
Marshfield Clinic, Wis.

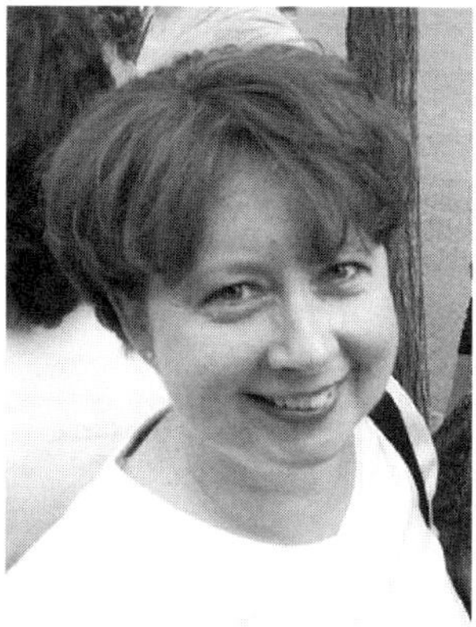

Chapter Ten

Moving Forward

By Amy White, Tomah, Wis.

I was diagnosed with breast cancer for the first time in the fall of 2003. I had just turned 37. The insanity of the next three years of my life began that July. I had been sitting on my couch watching TV when I scratched an itch near my left breast. In doing so, I thought I felt a small lump. At first, I thought hmmm… no big deal probably a swollen gland, pimple or ingrown hair and promptly tried to put it out of my mind. But I kept coming back to it over the next couple of weeks to check to see if it was still there. It was. This was particularly frightening for me as I have a family history of breast cancer. My mother had been diagnosed in 1998 at the age of 52. She had two lumpectomies and radiation. My grandmother was diagnosed in the late 1970s, around the age of 56, and then again in 1997 when she was 76 years old. In both cases she had a mastectomy followed by radiation. There is no way to know if my great-grandmother would have developed breast cancer as she died when my grandmother was five, but there was talk that my grandma's maternal aunt had breast cancer.

It was because of this family history that I had asked my mom years earlier how I would know the difference between an ordinary lump and a cancerous lump. She said the more I did the self-breast exams on a regular basis, the more familiar I would be with my body. It is because of those words that I followed my intuition and went to her with my concerns. She encouraged me to see a doctor, which I did. Due to the family history, I was referred for a mammogram and ultrasound with the radiologist. However, I wasn't able to get in for 11 days and the stress of waiting was difficult. At first the appointment was fairly optimistic but as I watched the radiologist's face as he read my films, his brow line pulled together, he started to frown, and his voice changed from being upbeat to one of guarded suspicion and concern. Before I knew it I was being referred for a biopsy. Again I found myself in this pattern of hurry up and wait because the earliest appointment I could get was in 13 days. Then I waited another week to get the results. By this time I was a nervous wreck from the procedures and unanswered questions. I tried to busy myself with my family and my job, but the fear was always hanging over me. Finally, my family doctor received the results and called me in to tell me I had cancer. It was official. My maternal medical history had caught up with me and I was now the third generation to be diagnosed with breast cancer. I thought I was going to faint. It was like a slap in the face, but in all honesty, one that my gut told me was coming. The events of the last four weeks led me to believe it was not going to be good news.

It's from this point that everything began to happen too fast. A couple of days later I was meeting with my surgeon. She discussed lumpectomy, mastectomy, sentinel nodes, axillary nodes, statistics, what the operation entailed and the recovery time. My head was whirling and I felt so overwhelmed. I could hardly concentrate on what was being said. I felt like I was sitting there nodding like one of those bobble head dolls. The next week I was meeting with my oncologist and radiation oncologist to go over potential treatment options, and by the end of the week I was in surgery. I had never been sick up to this point and the anxiety of surgery, needles, IV's, and dealing with cancer in general put me into panic attack mode. At this time, I opted for a lumpectomy. Later my test results confirmed a high grade infiltrating carcinoma, hormone negative, HER2-positive. It was decided that my treatment would include 12 weeks of chemotherapy (one treatment every third week) and radiation. Each chemo session lasted two to three hours.

My first chemotherapy appointment was the most terrifying experience of my life. I tried so hard to put on a brave face and a smile. To act like I could do this with some grace and dignity, but my body betrayed me again. I dreaded the insertion of the IV's, I dreaded knowing that my body was going to be pumped full of poison, I dreaded the possibility of the chemo making me sick, I dreaded the idea of losing my hair, and I dreaded the idea of my family seeing me in this vulnerable state. The fear swallowed me up and I passed out. When I came to I was laying in a recliner with my husband holding a cold compress on my forehead. That following afternoon and evening I was sicker than I had ever imagined I could be. I didn't eat for three days after my chemo, but when I was ready I could literally eat a 16 oz. steak, baked potato, vegetables and a big glass of water. Then half an hour later I would be ready to eat a Big Mac and a chocolate shake.

As I faced cancer, I found out fast that it invades one's life on a variety of different levels. It's not just a person's physical well-being that is affected but also the mental and emotional aspects as well. When I was first diagnosed, I just wanted to go inside my house, close the door and not come out until it was all over. In addition, cancer doesn't just attack the individual -- it attacks the whole family. It undermines everyone's sense of well-being and security, especially the children. The word cancer for me invoked fear. Fear of the unknown path I was suddenly forced to walk and yes, fear of death. How can the "D" word not be a concern when you have been diagnosed? I often looked at my children and wondered; will I see my son graduate, will I be there to help my daughter get ready for the prom, what about my husband or my parents and the rest of my family? I worried about our finances and how we were going to pay the bills. I worried about what my insurance would cover and how much. As I slowly began to process what was happening to me, I began to read and ask more questions. This was my way of taking some control back. My oncologist prescribed medication to help me manage the anxiety and nausea and was available to answer any question or concern I had.

But then the hair started to fall out. After my husband brought me home from my first treatment I found myself constantly checking my hair. I kept telling myself it's not a big deal, its only hair. I'm not the first or last woman to endure this and I will get through it. But as hard as I tried to brace myself for the inevitable, I knew I would never be ready. It was times like these that I wished I was stronger. That I could be like some movie star woman who shaved her head to play a part in a movie and have the self-confidence, self-assurance, and self-esteem to face the world. It is simply amazing how a little thing like hair can bring you to your knees. I am not a vain woman but this was one more example of the lack of control. The fact that I couldn't do anything to stop it -- and it wasn't enough that I was sick on the inside, I would now look sick on the outside. As my hair began to thin out, it actually itched and ached. I needed to make a decision, was I going to take control and cut my hair first or was I going to let cancer take a little more each day? As much as I psyched myself up for this moment, nothing prepared me for seeing myself in the mirror for the first time. I went from having shoulder length hair to listening to the shears leaving me a little more than an inch of hair on my head. I tried hard to keep it all in perspective but I worried about what my husband was thinking and feeling. Would he still find me attractive? Lord knows I didn't feel attractive.

The further I got into my chemo treatments, the more fatigue and mood swings I experienced. The rest of my hair had fallen out by now and I didn't even recognize the person looking back in the mirror. I found it difficult to wear caps and wigs all the time. They itched and irritated my head after a while. I had some bad days in which I began to question all over again why this was happening and I cried a lot. I usually saved my tears for the shower, or when I knew I was alone so that no one would be able to see or hear me. I was just so tired of being tired, and tired of not having control of my life. In a nutshell, I was tired of having cancer. I finally reached this point where I told myself that I needed to toughen up, focus and be positive. I would be alright and I would get through this. I reminded myself how blessed I was to have such a supportive family and an incredible group of co-workers and friends.

To help keep some normalcy in our home, my daughter and I put the Christmas tree up early. I was scheduled to have my next chemo appointment the day before Thanksgiving and traditionally we always put our tree up that following weekend. It was important to me to keep as many routines as possible to help the kids feel more secure. Throughout this ordeal, my husband and I were always honest with our kids about my illness. If they had questions or concerns we answered them as honestly as we could. Though we may not have always provided them with all the details, we felt that it was very important to talk to them openly about the cancer rather than let them hear whispered bits and pieces. This approach helped to give them some reassurance that I was doing OK. I also made it a priority to speak with my grandma as often as possible and let her know how I was. My being diagnosed a second time was especially hard on her and she often blamed herself for both my mom and I having cancer. I remember talking with her many times trying to comfort her and ease her fears, as well as her tears.

In December 2003, I received my last chemo treatment. I was very sick afterwards but I was thankful it was over. A month later, I started my radiation treatments. I went everyday, Monday through Friday, for 33 treatments. By the end of February 2004, I had completed my therapies and was back to work full-time. Everything looked great and my prognosis was very positive. My family began to heal and created a routine in which we put the last year behind us and looked forward to new beginnings.

But then 10 months later, during a routine mammogram the radiologist found a suspicious area in my right breast. She did everything she could to get a good picture of the area and a biopsy, but it was difficult because it was in such an odd spot. I was in shock and disbelief. I couldn't believe it was happening all over again. My kids were looking forward to that day as we were going to celebrate Christmas with my in-laws. Now I found myself in a situation that blindsided me big time.

The following week, I had a surgical lumpectomy with a wire localization to diagnose whether or not the area was cancerous. It was. During an exam, my surgeon also found a lump on my thyroid so I made an additional appointment to see a specialist and have it checked. (Thankfully those results came back negative.) We discussed the possible surgical options including mastectomy. The idea of this just about sent me over the edge. I was only 38. I had just jumped through all these hoops to get well. Why was this happening again? Afterwards, my surgeon sent me to the Mayo Clinic for a breast MRI to get a better idea of what we might be dealing with.

By now four weeks had passed since that day in December. Due to the stress, I lost close to 15 pounds. I went back to Mayo for my results and a second opinion. I remember distinctly being called to door "C." I remember that because as I walked up to the nurse I thought, "C" for cancer. I met with the doctors and the results of the MRI were not good. There was a suspicious spot on the left breast that I had the lumpectomy on and there were two areas in the right breast. Now I was faced with the agonizing decision of whether or not to have a bilateral mastectomy. As the doctors talked, I could see their mouths moving but I couldn't hear what they were saying. I was so devastated by the news that I just couldn't bring myself to focus on what they were trying to say to me. I was fortunate to have my aunt with me and she asked the questions that I either couldn't think to ask or just couldn't bring myself to ask. Now I needed to go home and tell my husband and my parents. I cried all the way home, much like I did when I was diagnosed the first time. Only now, cancer had really upped the ante.

I began to worry about everything from how this would affect the kids, to how were we going to pay the bills, what was I going to do about work when I had no sick leave left, to how will my husband cope and how would he feel about my appearance if I went through with the mastectomies. I also thought to myself what if this time I don't make it. We were just getting our lives back to normal and the bills paid off when cancer literally snuck up and ripped the carpet out from underneath us all. What was I going to do? For a while I wasn't so sure that I had the strength within me to pick myself up.

After much soul searching and a special talk with an incredible lady about her experience with bilateral mastectomies and reconstructive surgery, I chose the same. Signing the surgical authorization paper was one of the hardest things I have ever done. In my mind, I was still confused as to how things got so out of control. I did everything I was supposed to.

In February 2005, I had my surgery and stayed longer in the hospital than anticipated due to a complication with my port. It nicked part of my lung and as a result I had difficulty breathing. My surgeon promptly inserted a chest tube and it took several days for my lung to heal. In the meantime, my mother stayed in the hospital with me. I can only imagine how difficult all of this has been for my mother and father. Parents want to be able to shield their children, regardless of their age, from all the bad things. They want to be able to fix whatever is wrong. But in this case, it wasn't an option. I can't begin to understand the level of helplessness they must have felt having to watch from the sidelines.

It took awhile before I was able to look at myself in the mirror. Seeing myself with drains and expanders from the first phase of the reconstruction was overwhelming. Eventually, I took that step and moved on. Though there was no cancer found on my left side, my pathology report came back indicating both a high grade infiltrating carcinoma, hormone positive and HER2-negative, and the second spot was a lobular cancer. So in my mind, I knew that I had made the right decision regarding the mastectomies. Each week I met with my plastic surgeon who continued the expansion process. I was able to do this at the same time I was receiving chemotherapy. The decision to have a port put in was a good one. Though there were some difficult times accessing it, it was much easier than having my arms poked each week for 12 weeks.

During this time, I also came to terms with what was happening to me. It is what it is and no amount of crying, obsessing, feeling sorry for myself or being angry would change that. I decided nothing less than a positive attitude was acceptable. In order to take control I looked for ways to educate myself about my situation. You know what they say -- knowledge is power. I learned to laugh more and find humor in dealing with my cancer. I made an effort not to isolate myself from the friends and family that loved me. I tried to make going to chemotherapy a party. I brought music, food, cheese trays, books, magazines and my aunt. You never knew what she was going to say next, so that in itself was an adventure. The nurses often closed the door and I'm still not sure if that was for our privacy or because we were loud, and at times, a little on the rowdy side. By empowering myself, I believe that not only helped my physical well-being, but helped towards healing me emotionally. I'm not saying I never had a bad day. I did slip once in awhile, like the day that I lost my hair for the second time. But I overcame it and continued on. There were many days to look forward to, like when my final reconstructive surgery was completed.

To bring awareness and information that might be helpful to my sister, our daughters and my brother's daughter, I met with a genetic counselor. Based on the family information I was able to give him, he used modeling software that predicted a greater than 90% probability that I would likely be found to carry some kind of BRCA gene mutation. However, when the results came back they were inconclusive. What does this mean? It could mean a couple of things, but more than likely it means that I do have some kind of genetic predisposition, but at this time, the specific gene involved is unidentifiable. The testing also allowed me to be proactive in guarding against the possibility of ovarian cancer.

I discussed the results with my oncologist and he agreed that being proactive would be a good idea. I had a blood test which came back negative and in February of 2006 I had an ultrasound. The test found that I had a suspicious spot on my left ovary. The characteristics that the spot was exhibiting indicated that it could be cancerous. This again was another hard time for both myself and my family. I had read about ovarian cancer and I knew that it could be quite nasty. Again I was scared, but I prepared myself for round three. I met with the doctor a week later and she explained what my surgical options were. Going in I had made up my mind that I would have a complete abdominal hysterectomy. At times, I felt like cancer was taking bits and pieces of me a little at a time, but then again, I thought if cancer is coming back for me I was not going to lay down and go quietly. I was going to fight. The day I met with the doctor, my aunt went with me and I said to her, "Do you know where I was a year ago today?" She said, "No, where were you?" I replied, "Upstairs having my mastectomies."

Shortly thereafter I had my surgery and my husband was able to get the preliminary results. The doctor told him it was not cancer. For a man that had said very little about my health, he finally broke down and cried. I woke up several hours later in the same room that

I was in when I had my mastectomies. The first question I asked was if it was cancer. My husband told me no. I just couldn't believe it. There had been so much bad news over the past couple of years that I had to keep asking over and over to let it sink in. We were so relieved and grateful.

My experience with cancer has taught me so much. If I were to share any words of encouragement for women currently facing cancer it would be these. Find a doctor(s) that you are comfortable with, who, you feel, listens to your questions and concerns. We have some incredible doctors, nurses and healthcare professionals out there -- it's just a matter of finding the right one for you. Once you are ready to start processing what is happening to you, become your own advocate. Educate yourself about your cancer and don't be afraid to ask questions. Write down what you want or need to ask prior to meeting with the doctor, or take someone with you to your appointments to help you remember what was said. Take an active role in your healthcare by asking for copies of your test results, learning to read a pathology report and knowing what medications you are taking, why you are taking them and the dosage.

Keep a journal of your experiences. Cancer is not just physical, it is emotional, and there are some thoughts and emotions that need to be expressed. Writing can help to heal by validating your feelings. Remember it is OK to cry. Being positive 24/7 and wearing a reassuring smile for the benefit of others can be extremely exhausting. Crying can be a release from the frustration and the fear. Let the people who love you help you. As much as you may want to continue to handle this on your own, family and friends are also struggling. People genuinely want to help but may be unsure as to what to do. A wonderful friend once told me not to be afraid of the love and support and to accept the help in the spirit in which it is given. I found out that this love and support was perhaps, the best "medicine" of all.

Finally, what is the most important lesson cancer has taught me? Cancer has taught me to slow down, enjoy my family, and each day that God has given me. I'm getting better at rolling with the punches, accepting change and not sweating the small stuff. Cancer has taught me that I am stronger than I gave myself credit for. That despite the challenges, I am a fighter, and that cancer can't keep this good woman down. Cancer has taught me to live my life in the present and to concentrate on what is in front of me, not behind me. Cancer has taught me that I have a lot to share and I know now that I would love the opportunity to use my educational background and experience to help other women find their way. Cancer has taught me to take that leap of faith and live life to the fullest. To step outside what is comfortable and routine and open myself up to new experiences and projects. A positive and assertive attitude, excellent healthcare workers, my faith, and the incredible love and support of family and friends are what really helped to move me forward. As traumatic as the cancer diagnoses were, in a strange and ironic twist, it also turned out to be a gift. Maybe now I am beginning to understand what the phrase "God has a plan for you" means.

Women who have mutations in the BRCA1 or BRCA2 genes have a significantly increased risk to develop ovarian cancer. If your family is considering testing for BRCA1/2, it is best to test a person affected with breast/ovarian cancer first.

- Christina Zaleski, MS, CGC, Senior Genetic Counselor, Marshfield Clinic, Wis.

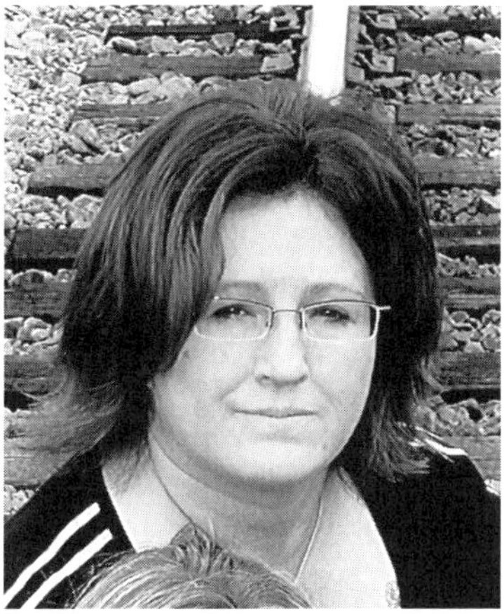

Chapter Eleven

Here for the Fight

By Rose Storkel, Norwalk, Wis.

My first experience with breast cancer was when I was 10. I developed an opinion at an early age about what I would do if I ever got breast cancer. I decided that after watching what the chemo did to my mother, I would rather die than go through that. I'm 42 now and I've pretty much felt the same for all these years. I was in denial about what it would mean if it ever really happened to me.

That day came in late August of 2006. After years of missing my mammogram appointments and sloppily performing self-breast exams, I felt a lump in my left breast. By the grace of God, something told me this needed my attention. My husband, Buck, was relentless about me going in to have it checked out. When I saw my doctor, he asked, "What do you think?" My response was immediate, "I think it's something." We agreed it would be best to get that mammogram I had put off for three years.

I went to La Crosse, Wis. that Friday. What began as a mammogram progressed into needing more films on my left breast, then an ultrasound and finally a biopsy. After I saw the films from the mammogram, I knew it was serious. To me it looked something like I had always feared – a dark area on the film. The doctor who performed the biopsy confirmed my fear. She said, "You have breast cancer." I asked how she knew and she said, "I've been doing this for 20 years – it didn't move." The tumor she was referring to had two dark areas; we didn't know whether it was one tumor or two.

My mother, whom I referred to earlier, is a 32-year survivor. She was at every appointment with me from the very first. She was there that day, and when I left the doctors office and found her, we held each other and cried. I called and talked to my kids and my husband and cried some more. I didn't know what to think, I was in shock.

Something happened that day that helped me decide that I wasn't going to die. I think if I hadn't had the experience I did, I may not have had the same attitude going through this whole thing. My mom said she had been at a garage sale earlier that day and the lady had some beautiful jewelry. I wanted to go look. When we got there, the gal looked just awful. She explained that her husband of 18 years had left her a note that he was leaving her for another woman. My thoughts took me back to when I experienced the pain of divorce. I knew immediately that this was the worst pain I had ever been through, and I would not trade my news for the news she had gotten. I bought a blue sapphire ring, which I only took off for my surgery. The ring is an inspiration to me and makes me think of the day I decided to live – not to let this cancer beat me.

Seeing a surgeon was the next step, and I feel very lucky to have met the surgeon that would take care of me. Every time she had bad news -- I could tell as she slid the folder across the table -- she cared how it was going to affect me. She always started out by saying, "I'm sorry, it's not good news."

I had a type three out of four cancer and there were some decisions to be made. I still wish to this day that they could just take the cancer out and you didn't have to be the one to decide. I could have a lumpectomy and radiation, have one breast removed, or opt to have both breasts removed. There were a lot of factors involved with whatever I decided. It didn't take long to decide that the best course for me would be to have both breasts removed and have the reconstructive surgery. My mother never had any reconstruction done and I knew that I didn't want to live the rest of my life without breasts.

My next appointment was with a plastic surgeon. He explained what we could do to reconstruct my breasts. The reconstruction would start the day of surgery, there were spacers that would be put in after the breasts were removed. After I was through with my chemo, they would reconstruct the nipple and areola and put in an implant.

Everything happened very quickly and the next week I was waking up after the surgery. I looked down and I already had new breasts; that was the best thing for me. I probably didn't have to experience the loss some women feel because they were not completely gone. I tried to think that I was just getting new breasts; some women do it by choice.

I have the best husband in the world, he has been honest about his feelings throughout everything and he spent every moment with me in the hospital. I couldn't have handled the aftercare with emptying the drains and bandaging myself. He got up every morning and took care of me before going to work. You really know you are loved when someone can tell you that as long as you are smiling, that's all that matters. He held me when I cried out of frustration. When I lost my hair we both found humor in making jokes about my wig, calling it my muskrat. He called me "skin" and it always made me smile. Some people thought it wasn't funny, but we did, and that was all that mattered.

I have had some great support from my family, especially my mom, Sharon, and my cousin, Gail, who called me constantly to be sure I was OK. My kids, Jeremy and Kristen, have had their ups and downs with this, but I can only imagine how scary it is for them.

When my mother had cancer, I remember going to doctor's appointments with her. Back then, all of the cancer patients were all together. We would go to the hospital for appointments and I remember a long hall that everyone who had cancer of any type would sit and wait. Some people didn't have noses or ears or couldn't talk because they had their voice box removed. It was terrifying to see and I would think that we were lucky not to have something like that. My mom was very strong and didn't ever let on if she thought she wasn't going to survive.

We didn't talk about cancer at our house. I wasn't even sure what my mom had, I just knew she had been crying and throwing up a lot. There were a lot of doctor's appointments. I did see her changing clothes once, she had a very big sore area, and what I thought looked like a cave in her chest. My brother and I just did whatever we could around the house to make things easier for her. She didn't feel well for most of the first year or so of her fight. This was a very hard time for our family, but I'm sure it prepared me a little for what I had coming.

Having my mother still here after 32 years almost took the fear in some way out of my prognosis. I don't think anyone could have made me believe that I too, wasn't going to beat this. Mom never seemed to feel she wasn't going to win and I never heard her say she was giving up. I know that having the attitude that you are going to make it is the best medicine you can take.

The first thing I checked out was how my insurance would take care of this and if I would be covered. The second thing I did was go to work and let them know what I was going through. I work at Jellystone Park in Warrens, Wis. as a retail manager. When I went to my boss about my illness, I was told not to worry about anything whatsoever. I was allowed to work anytime I felt like I could come to work. I know how rare this is and how fortunate I am to have an employer like Ed Vandermolen to work for. It's such an unreal experience to know there are people that just care about you as a person, not a body showing up to work everyday.

I met LeRoy Butler through his work here at Jellystone Park. LeRoy has been to the park many times raising money for his Foundation. I never thought I would be one of the people being helped out by the Foundation though. As soon as he found out that someone at the park had breast cancer, he was offering to let me apply for help, if needed. Things were difficult for us because I was not working very many hours, if any at all. I was blessed with some support, but I think the best part of meeting LeRoy was the look in his eyes when I first met him, and the words of support he gave me and my family that day. He is the real deal and his heart is genuine.

The day I met the other ladies in this book was the first time I had been around other people going through the same thing that I was. That day I was the most comfortable that I had been in a long time, because I knew they were going through, or had gone through, the very same things. I felt comfortable because they aren't people on the outside of this telling you what to do. They have had to make all the choices themselves. There is a comfort in knowing that they have had this experience. Just like the feeling like I have with my mom, she tries to explain to my children what I'm going through. She knows -- but hopefully they will never have to know. It's also an honor to be with ladies who are so courageous and will continue the fight for themselves and others.

Overall though, I did feel that the other ladies thought I hadn't had cancer long enough to fully know what I was talking about. That could be true -- I guess only time will tell. I do know that I have a lot of years to experience what this will mean for me, my family, and my friends, and I'm thankful for that.

The reality of that day with everyone was that all of us aren't going to make it. This disease will take some of these beautiful people from us. Some of their struggles will be enormous. It has great meaning for me; it will forever impact my life to have had a chance to be part of such a special group of women who will fight to help others when they need so much themselves.

I have just finished my reconstructive surgery and I must say that it isn't the same as having what you once had, but it definitely beats having nothing. I realized when I met the other women that day that this procedure isn't for everyone. Mom and I sat at breakfast with two other ladies who had breast cancer and it was not for them, they were very opposed to it. I very much respect that. In retrospect, there are so many choices we each have to face in the process, and we will each do what is right for us. Each time I was faced with a choice it's been torture for me. I wished each time that someone else would just make it, but all you can do is get your options, talk to your family and friends, get their opinion, and then ultimately it's up to you.

My prognosis is good and my attitude will continue to be good as well. I'm part of a special group; some of these special people won't win the battle, but we're here for the fight.

Insurance coverage for the cost of normal health care related to participating in a clinical trial is now mandated in Wisconsin. AB617 (2006), Act 194 was passed in March 2006 and went into effect Nov. 1, 2006. Wisconsin is one of about half of the states across the nation that have enacted such a law, following Medicare's lead that mandated coverage since 2000. To learn more about insurance coverage related to clinical trials go to www.ncsl.org/programs/health/clinicaltrials.htm, or www.cancer.gov/clinicaltrials/digestpage/medicare, or www.cancertrialshelp.org/patientsCaregivers/insurance.jsp, or do a web search on your own to gain information.

- Kim Fuehrer, RN, BSN, MSM, Oncology Administrative Specialist, Marshfield Clinic, Wis.

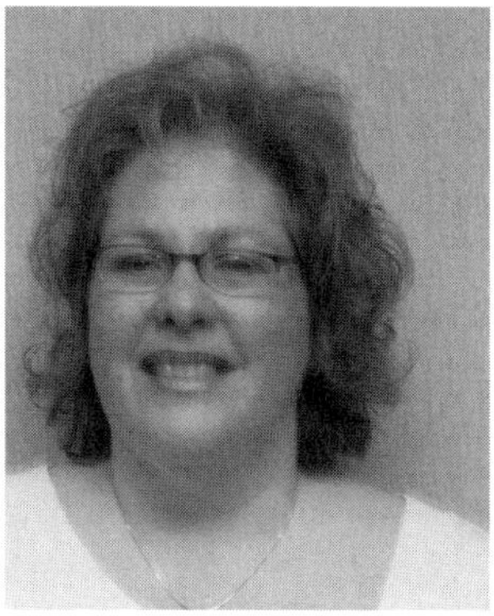

Chapter Twelve

Leap of Faith of Women

By Heidi Schoenberger, Beaver Dam, Wis.

Approximately three years ago I became tired all the time. My body ached. I went to the doctor and he told me I was anemic. So I started more iron. It did not help. I began forgetting things – the days of the week, my boys' names, appointments, entering things into the checkbook, and a few times walking out of stores without paying for things. My blood work showed I was B12 deficient, so I began injections. My husband, Eric, and teenage son, Nick, gave them to me. We also have an autistic 9-year old, Spencer, that our teen helps with. This did not seem fair for my teenager to have to help out so much, yet he never complained. I began having pain under my left rib. It was sharp and painful. The surgeon knew it was not a hernia, but did not know what it was, so he continued to inject it with cortisone to numb the pain. It helped for about one month, but came right back.

I was later told that the first symptoms of my illness were tiredness, anemia, pale skin and swollen spleen, right where my pain was. This was missed. I am 44 years old and just had my 45th surgery.

Then I began to catch anything people around me had. Cold, flu, bronchitis, and pneumonia. I was treated for each one, just to have it return again. I had to quit my job over three years ago. I was just too ill to know if I could make it to work the next day. I began having blood transfusions, and this would help for about two weeks and then I would feel tired again. Our family has been struggling financially and I feel to blame.

After having pleurisy (an infection around the lining of the lungs) for the fourth time in a row, the ER doctor ran more tests and found out that I have Chronic Myeloid Leukemia (C.M.L.). At first I misunderstood and thought, "OK, so they will give me a pill (added to the huge list I now take) and I will be all better." Two days later I saw an oncologist. He told me I would have my blood drawn weekly, that they would watch me closely, and that I would start a new medication. I walked out the door and the nurse gave me a bouquet of daffodils. I wondered how she knew my birthday was just five days away. I thanked her and was so surprised when she said, "This is for a ray of hope." I asked what I needed a ray of hope for. She replied, "Heidi, do you understand that you have cancer?"

I felt like my world crashed before me. No one had mentioned the "C" word to me. Now I understood why my husband shed tears in the ER just two nights before. The next day I received a package from the American Cancer Society. It was a wig. I said no way am I having this. I will let go and let God. I would not do all that horrible chemo and radiation stuff, not me, no way. I draw the line here! This is not happening to me. Not after all I have been through so far. My family needs me.

It is amazing the emotions one goes through -- denial, shock, fear, depression, anger and finally acceptance. This is when I knew I had to learn more about leukemia. God was telling me to slow down. To listen to my aching body and take care of it. Don't push it. I asked questions – lots of questions. Sometimes I liked the answers, but most of the time I did not. For example, the cure for leukemia is a bone marrow transplant. It is best to use one of your siblings as a donor. Two of my four brothers were willing. The sibling who is the farthest in age is the best to choose. One should also have a transplant before they are 50 years of age. However, the donor has to match in five categories. This does not often happen. Also, the person needing the transplant has to be strong enough. Because I have asthma, weak lungs and poor kidneys, I am not a candidate. The end – I cannot have a bone marrow transplant. I hate road blocks.

March 2006

Thought I would keep a journal on my cancer. Went to the ER with what I thought was pleurisy again; I had it last month and the December before. After the chest x-ray and the doctors trying three pain meds in my IV to no relief, a different doctor came in and did some blood work. He found my white blood count at 65,000. Normal is 3,000. A bit high. He told me not to worry; all I needed was more blood transfusions like last year. No worries. I saw an oncologist who lost his wife to cancer and he told me I had Chronic Myeloid Leukemia. Then he walked out of the room. I was to see him next week. He comes from our state capitol, Madison, Wis., every Tuesday to treat cancer patients.

I met with the doctor again and he told me two choices. One, do chemo for two months -- if I do not reject it. He has three other types to try, each one with more horrible side effects. Then do radiation on my whole body to kill all of my cancerous bone marrow. The number one choice would be my siblings' bone marrow for a complete transplant. My oldest brother volunteered. If the marrow transplant takes, I live – if not, I die -- because all of my marrow is now gone. Choice number two was what I chose – take chemo and hope I do not reject it, I have again up to three types to try, each one having worse side effects. He is hoping to "buy" me two to three years. Before I am 50 years old (I just turned 44), I must have a transplant. My brother would then be 60 years old.

Smile – it gets better! The meds are expensive he tells me. So I go to the pharmacy. They say, "I'm sorry Heidi, we cannot fill this prescription." I ask why and they say, "We do not do transactions over $1,000. This medication is $10,000 for 30 days." I was to start the meds yesterday. What to do? My chest and back pain are almost unbearable. I will go into the hospital again tonight.

March 31, 2006

At $36 per pill, I'm having to be like a baby bird and hold my mouth up into the air, and as I vomit swallow it again so I don't lose the pill. Not fun. My face has a "masking" where it has turned red and sore as if I have been sun burned. It is hot and itches and feels like little blisters. I still have hair and it has been 12 days on chemo. Cross your fingers! I did have to get a bonnet to keep the sun off of my face. Since I had my blood drawn again at nine days after starting chemo, my white blood cells dropped from 65,000 to 50,000. I thought this was good, the doctor said not good enough. It is going slow. He had decided to do the bone marrow transplant this fall instead of in two years. I am continuing to get sick. The doctor thinks it's the chemo. I think it is the antinausea meds. The morphine is very drugging. It does take the edge off though.

Spencer is having a difficult time that I am not able to play with him. The doctor wants me to drop the chemo (Gleevec) to just one time per day and he will call in a new nausea med.

April 3, 2006

I hurt so bad. Every muscle in my body aches. Nothing seems to help the pain but two morphine, which I cannot take and watch Spencer. I am looking into every resource of respite for Spencer that I can find. This is so unfair to him. He likes the idea of daycare and summer camp. I'll keep working on that.

April 4, 2006

Still hurting today. Slept well this morning on morphine. Went to the doctor, he wants to stop the chemo for a week to see for sure if that is what's causing all of my muscle and joint pain, or is it arthritis? He is now concerned that I would not be a good candidate for radiation, not that he is ruling it out, but because if I am having such a hard time on the Gleevec, how would I handle radiation

April 9, 2006

The lab made an error and used the wrong tubes to draw my blood, so I have to have it drawn again to look for internal bleeding. I will find out on Monday or Tuesday. I got to take a "drug vacation" -- a break from the chemo. The first morning I could move my arms. I felt great. Each day off of chemo I feel better, yet I know next Tuesday I go back on it. I will be a on a lower dose and he will help me try to ease the pain with meds. The blood tests did show that I went from 69,000 white blood cells to 14,000, so it helped lots. I expect it to go up after being off for a week, but it works and it is helping. I do not go through radiation until my blood level is at 5,000 or less. The side effects suck – well, so does cancer!

<u>May 6, 2006</u>

I went to the oncologist and my blood level was now 8,000. He said that we are ready to set up an appointment with the transplant people in Madison. I'm waiting to hear on that. Once my levels are between 3,000 and 5,000, I am ready for radiation and a transplant. Then I will be cross-typed, matched, and see if my older brothers are a match. I do not feel as tired or weak, but still need to not overdo it.

<u>May 31, 2006</u>

I met the doctor in Madison, Wis. He's a very nice doctor in his mid-30s and he knows leukemia well. He looked at how fast my white blood cells dropped and even though this seemed very good, he is concerned that they may bottom out and then go real high again. Another concern is that my red blood cells still say that I am anemic. Also the fact that I have kidney problems and do not have a good set of lungs is making me not a good candidate for a bone marrow transplant. My spleen is still enlarged. So all my worry has been put on the back burner.

The bad part is that there is no alternative for me. If my counts go so high again, and the Gleevec is not controlling it, all I can do is buy time and hope that one of the two new possible chemo meds that are in the process of being approved, are approved and I accept them. It was a long day. He told me to continue on with my claim for disability, he said I will remain tired and most likely not be able to keep a job. Every three weeks I will have a blood draw from my local doctor and every three months have a very detailed blood draw in Madison -- unless things get worse before then. Depending on my levels in six months, or in March, he will do a bone marrow draw from my back hip area and read things then.

July 12, 2006

Went to my new oncologist. Very nice, he comes from Madison and takes my insurance. He has cut me a deal. As long as I promise to have my blood drawn every two weeks and the levels stay, level, I can hold off on the chemo. If I have trouble, then I have to go back on. Fair to me!

July 15, 2006

I feel horrible. I thought it was just a cold, but I cannot produce a good cough. It's stuck. I cannot breathe and I'm dizzy and confused. I have been trying the over the counter expectorant with no avail. I have been doing my duo nebs at home with no relief. Off to the ER. The temp is 108 outside. The air conditioning does not even help. From the house, to the van, to the hospital, I almost stopped breathing. As soon as I entered the hospital, the nurses put me in a wheelchair and took me in front of all others. They gave me an epinephrine injection and oxygen, duo nebs, IV's and prednisone, which I hate; it makes me feel so crappy. They did chest x-rays and found pneumonia. Finally three days later I was beginning to feel a bit better and went off the oxygen and prednisone. I begged the doctor because it makes me feel so bad. Then I have to have three cavities fixed. I got three migraines. I think it was from the prednisone. So now I was taking meds to stop the migraines.

July 18, 2006

I'm so dizzy and feel terrible. I think I have a sinus infection. I have a headache and drainage down the back of my throat. My ears feel achy, and my glands, too. I had to have my eyes examined today and with the chemo damage, I have to get new glasses. My sight is so blurry. This happens the doctor said, as well as the sores in my mouth. This is so fun and it is so hot outside!

July 21, 2006

Went to the doctor's office. Blood test showed that my white cells are rising. However, he is letting me go on vacation to the trip we won to the Bahamas for a week, and then I start meds when I return.

July 23, 2006

I became very ill in Bahamas with itching, red rash, hives and spleen pain. The jet landed and I was taken to the hospital over night with an ear infection, prednisone for the hives, ear drops and an antibiotic. I was also sun burned. I felt terrible and weak. After I was quarantined for two days, I am still on high doses of prednisone, Gleevec for the cancer and meds to boost the chemo and lower my high white blood cells. I run a low grade temp and always feel hot from the prednisone or the temp. At least the ear infection and hives are better. I see the doctor on Sept. 9. I sure feel better with a little brown on my skin!

Sept. 11, 2006

Today I had a titanium med port put into my chest surgically. Now I can have blood draws, IVs and medication put directly into my port because my veins have all collapsed. My chest and shoulder are tender red and bruised. In 10 days my stitches should be healed and today we went to the hematologist and bone marrow transplant specialist. Because of my health, I would still be a very poor candidate for a transplant. The meds are not bringing my white blood cell count down. He is starting me on Sprycel. At this time it is the last hope for a cure for me. Another med is coming out next year. It is not FDA approved yet. I could maybe go to Illinois state to stay for trial, but I don't want to miss the boys or Eric.

Oct. 1, 2006

The pain my body is experiencing is horrible. At first I get a headache and blurred vision. I feel like I am in slow motion. My legs below the knees feel like a tight rubber band is cutting off circulation. I try to walk and the pain between my head, legs, back and knees is horrible. My hips often hurt as well. It seems worse after I rest. Yet I need to rest or my back and mind tire so easily. I'm taking longer naps now. I have diarrhea and stomach cramps. I am usually only hungry once a day. I'm depressed and I cannot do what I once did, and am missing out on things. I have to plan things that I really want to do and accept if I cannot go. I got a cane because I almost fell face first on a staircase.

Oct. 10, 2006

I saw my bone marrow, transplant and hematologist doctor today. He did lots of blood work. My white cells are at 11. The normal is 14, but it was better than last week before I had my blood transfusion. I was at 8.2, way too low. I had two units of blood and seven hours later was sent home. I was exhausted. Before, whenever I had a transfusion, I felt like a million bucks, not this time. He was going to start me on injections bi-weekly to bring my blood cells up. He will wait until he sees my labs in two weeks, but believes that my levels will drop again and that they are up just because I had a transfusion last week. I will start the injections then.

<u>November 2006</u>

We started packing because we needed to sell our house. We could no longer afford the payments and insurance and need to find something that will cost us less.

We sold our house! We have 19 days to move. They wanted the day before Thanksgiving but we said no. We were moving until 12:30 Thanksgiving night. Eric broke down and cried. He felt that what I had prayed for – our house to sell, to move to one level and to get him and Spencer settled was coming true – and then I was going to give up on life. Then we had to take him to the ER, we were not sure if he was having a stroke, heart attack or anxiety. It turned out to be anxiety; he had not slept for nights and felt that I was not helping him. The hospital gave him meds to sleep and he did – like a rock. Woke up and we signed over our old house and put a down payment on our new house.

<u>December 2006</u>

Went to a Christmas party and met a man with C.M.L., like I have. Finally someone with the same leukemia. However, our side effects are so different and so is our treatment. He's doing much better than I did on my first chemo. My second chemo seems to be helping with fewer side effects than the first. My blood counts seem to be stabilizing more. The doctor said this is not remission as I had hoped. I have to go five years with no regressions.

Since I was diagnosed in March of 2006, new medications have come out to help leukemia patients. Not me, but some. I will not give up. I want to see my children marry and I want to become a grandmother. I want to retire with the loving husband the Lord gave me. So I am now on my second chemo. The first did not keep my levels down. It cost $10,000 per month. I have been on my second chemo just two weeks now. It's only $4,000 per month, besides all my other med's, labs and hospital and doctors bills. I really do not know how much I owe, but it's in the hundred thousands. Our insurance card ran out last week at the pharmacy, we had maxed out for the year. I have nine prescriptions waiting for me and no money for co-pays. So yes, we do have insurance, but it does not pay for everything. Many new experimental drugs are not covered. If I were to try the new one my doctor wants next, I would have to stay in Illinois for the study. I cannot do this with a family that needs me.

When people heard of my leukemia, they began praying for me. I go to a cancer support group. I am the youngest person in the group and the only person with leukemia. At first I felt out of place because leukemia is much different than "other cancers," but we always say a prayer at the end of the group. We are all in the same boat. The people in the group make me feel very welcome. It helps me to talk about my cancer. I appreciate each and every day. Truly. Just close your eyes and imagine that you have cancer. What does it mean to you or to your family and your loved ones? Be kind to one another. We never know what our neighbor, or their family, is going through.

Now try to open your eyes and wake up from this dream. I opened my eyes, but it wasn't a dream. I am so fortunate to have a wonderful church and Christian friends and the Lord above watching over me.

Update –

On Feb. 10, 2007, Eric, Heidi's husband, called the EMT's because Heidi had stopped breathing. On Valentine's Day, Heidi was released from the hospital and returned home with hospice care. Heidi was told that nothing could be done until the end.

Heidi Schoenberger passed away on May 5, 2007 at the age of 45.

My first reaction hearing about my only daughter's cancer was I would not believe it! I wouldn't talk about it. It is a complicated cancer to understand. We must work through this.

Heidi's father – Donald G. Hansen

When my daughter called and told me she was diagnosed with a blood cancer I was so angry at the very sound of this. She was crying so hard I felt I couldn't break down, too. I do this best by myself.

There were so many questions, and still are, why wasn't this found out before, because she has been so sick and can't keep up with things and been to so many doctors.

Heidi has three sons to think about and a wonderful husband – we will all have to work together. I am so proud of my sons to offer a bone marrow if it was possible (it is not advised).

Medicine is great – but all the prayers are so helpful!

Heidi's mother – Ramona J. Hansen

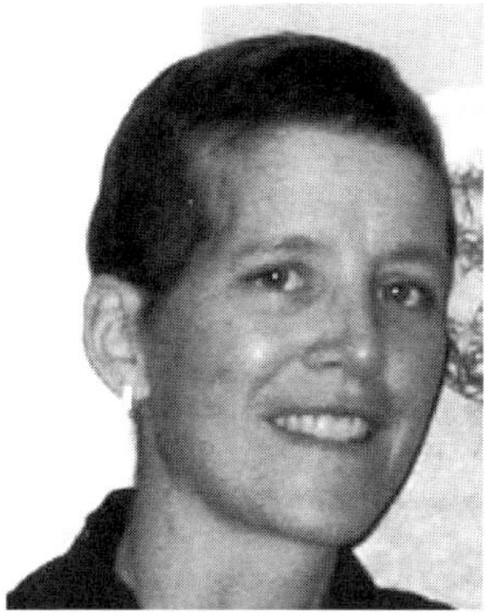

Chapter Thirteen

My Tribute to My Dear Friend: Shelly Duncan Bowman
By Deneen Pedersen, Tomah, Wis.

I had always told Shelly she should write a book about her experience with cancer. She would just laugh. Then LeRoy Butler was doing this book so I asked Shelly if she would do something for it. She said she didn't know what to say or how it would inspire others. I disagreed with her, because she had inspired me. She then agreed to do it as long as she had some help. Unfortunately she passed away before it could happen. Then LeRoy asked me to write about losing a dear friend to cancer.

Shelly and I met at age 10 and had been friends ever since. She succeeded in everything she did -- sports, academics and life in general. I always asked her how she did it all and her reply was, "I have fought for everything I have done." And she did. It didn't come naturally to her, but she worked hard for everything she did.

After graduation we had a circle of four friends that continued to see each other as we went on with our lives. We were there for each other through weddings, children and funerals. We made a pact to get together at least two times each year, to just catch up with each other. We lived in different towns and would travel to one of our homes to visit.

In 2001 everything changed with a phone call. Shelly was diagnosed with a brain tumor and the doctors had given her six months to live. I called our circle of friends to let them know. At that point, our circle grew stronger as our friendship needed to take this journey and support Shelly. Not being part of the family, we did not know all the details – we just knew that it was bad! I waited a few days then went to see Shelly in the hospital. I tried to think of some words of encouragement to give her and when I walked into the hospital room it was Shelly who gave me the words of encouragement.

She was going to "Kick Cancer's Butt." We talked together as we always did about future plans and family. Shelly was a fighter and she fought to live. Our circle of friends would get together every couple of months. As we saw her brain tumor get better, we were there to celebrate the big occasion. But soon after, breast cancer invaded her body – she lost both her breasts, did lots of chemo and radiation but always continued to encourage us that she was doing good. Throughout her six years of fighting breast cancer she was not willing to give up the fight. It was not up for discussion, the cure could be only a day away. Our goal during these special times together was for Shelly to not think about her cancer. When we got together there would only be a five minute discussion on how her cancer was doing. She always talked about the positive things that were happening to her body. They would find a new spot of cancer, but she would talk about an older spot that was now smaller. So the chemo and radiation was working and would work on this new spot also. The rest of the times together were talking about family, friends and future times together as we enjoyed a Dairy Queen Blizzard.

Shelly was always on the go. Not a day to waste or feel sorry for herself. Her worry was only for others -- her beautiful daughter, her loving husband and a great mom, dad, brother and many friends. Our small circle of friends were all turning 40 years old at the beginning of 2007. So we planned a mother–daughter trip to go to Florida and lie on a warm beach and celebrate. Two weeks before we were to leave on our trip, the cancer showed up throughout her body. Shelly would not be able to take the trip and had only a couple of weeks to live.

On my last trip to see Shelly, she was only worried about her family, and she introduced me to her wonderful doctor. We spent about 30 minutes talking about how to raise money for a hospice house in Eau Claire, Wis. I was shocked to find out a large city like Eau Claire did not have a hospice house. I have helped with many fund raisers and Shelly thought I could help. I hope to help in this event by bringing a Hospice House to Eau Claire.

Shelly Duncan Bowman died at home at the age of 40 years and 11 days. She kicked the cancer's butt for six years (five years, six months longer than expected). In those six years, Shelly lived a lifetime with family trips, time with her daughter and husband, special moments with family and taking a lot of walks with friends.

A week before Shelly's death I went to my doctor and she said she found a lump in my breast. I would need to have a mammogram. Funny part was, I was not as afraid as I thought I might be. I kept thinking about Shelly and knew I also could fight this if it came to that. I was one of the lucky ones and the mammogram came out good, but if it hadn't, I would hope that I would do Shelly proud and "Kick Cancer Butt" as each new day does bring a chance for a cure to be found.

I was honored that Shelly chose our circle of friends to be part of the pallbearers at her funeral. Our journey did not end as we put her casket in place to rest, but will continue as our circle of friends will continue to get together a couple times each year. And we know Shelly will be there with us – encouraging us, supporting us and watching over us, and I believe she will be enjoying the Dairy Queen Oreo Blizzard right along with us.

Shelly, I love you and miss you, but I know I will see you again.

Running so fast I can't feel my feet
It hurts to look back, so I keep my head straight
A light in the distance, it starting to fade
I run a bit faster, but the faster it fades
Closing my eyes, keep on going
Release the pain built inside
The tears start to roll but I can't stop to cry
Open my eyes, the light is gone
A sigh of relief fills the air
I turn to walk back, the light reappears.
Running so fast I can't feel my feet
It never stops, I run on repeat.

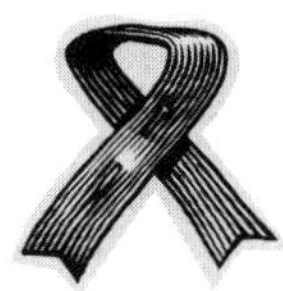

Let us all stand together and fight for each other
For our lives, and the lives of our friends
For the lives of our children, and our family so dear
We'll fight till the end, no matter how near
It may win some battles, but can't take the war
We have to keep fighting,
Hope it won't come back for more.
Pin on a ribbon, and don't give up.
I know it affects every one of us.
A great woman once said,
"Let's kick cancers butt"
So let's do as she said, and never give up
Cause we'll win the war
We'll win this war yet.
Just remember Shelly's words, and never forget.

-- Poems written by Tia Pedersen, age 15

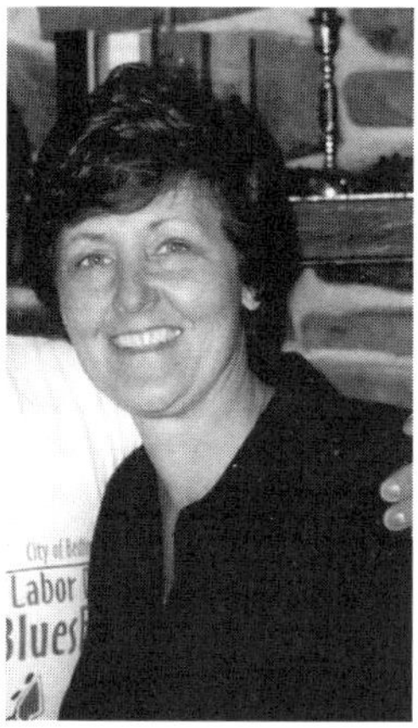

Chapter Fourteen

A Test of Faith

By Anne Jacobson, Wausau, Wis.

No words can adequately describe the feelings one has when she is told she has a rare form of cancer and it is serious… I was about to embark on the biggest life-changing and life-challenging circumstance in my life.

On Sept. 9, 2004, my uncle passed away after a 13-year fight with cancer. I remember talking with my brother while standing outside after his funeral. I told him, as I had watched the family respond to this crisis over many months, I could not imagine having cancer, and didn't know what I would do.

Two weeks later, on Sunday, Sept. 26, 2004, I awoke with a sharp pain in my left breast, which I immediately noticed was inflamed and swollen. The skin appeared striped and was definitely hot to the touch. My first thought as I stood in the shower was, "I have cancer. OK, Lord, we will deal with this together." I wondered if I should go to a walk-in clinic, but decided I would call my family physician first thing in the morning. I immediately started pondering the possible outcomes -- I had just turned 49 years old four days earlier. I had a husband and three children to care for. My sweet children were 20, 18 and 14. As this journey unfolded, they were each affected in unspoken, profound ways.

I called the clinic in the morning and was squeezed into the schedule, being seen by a physician assistant. She informed me that it appeared to be an infection. I was prescribed antibiotics and told to call in 48 hours if it had not resolved. The breast remained extremely painful and did not resolve. I continued to work and attempted to focus on the activities of everyday living. After arriving at work Wednesday morning, I called the doctor back and insisted on being seen. My gut told me this was serious. I returned to the clinic and my doctor appeared, gently announcing in a serious tone that she thought I had a rare form of breast cancer. This could only be confirmed through a biopsy, and she already had one scheduled for me that afternoon.

After the biopsy, I was advised it would be Monday morning, Oct. 4, before they would have the results. I appeared at 9 a.m. that morning, my husband in tow. He had been out of town the previous Monday, attending the funeral of his uncle who had died of cancer. When he returned, and I told him what was going on, he reacted with his usual rational, stoic manner. His strong demeanor is what would come to sustain me throughout my journey with this deadly disease. He never panicked, speculated, or became complaining. In other words, he was unchanging. But it was that strength of character for which I married him that would be invaluable to me and to our family in living with this challenge.

The surgeon advised I had "inflammatory breast cancer." I was told it was very serious and I needed to do something immediately. He actually walked us down the hall to the oncology department and introduced me to Dr. Steven Sorscher, the person whom I came to believe walked on water, and is an exceptional physician in many ways. He saw us immediately and explained the diagnosis and counseled us regarding its type and staging. I was told it was Stage III B. This didn't sound promising to me. When we asked what my prognosis was and what we should tell our children, we were advised that it was a rare, more aggressive form of breast cancer, representing about 1-2 percent of all breast cancers. I was told I had a 40 percent chance of being alive in five years. I had no high risk factors for contracting this disease. I told Dr. "S" then that if I was in the minority, I would be in the minority who survived this deadly disease! I asked him how soon we could start tackling this tumor -- he said there would be tests first, and we would start on Wednesday, since two of the tests could not be performed on the same day.

How could this be happening? My entire world was turned upside down in a minute. I was active and had always considered myself a healthy person. To this day, I have not been hospitalized, except to give birth. I had never had surgery before. The moment seemed surreal. In an instant, my priorities changed. Nothing seemed as important as tackling the challenge now set before me, and recovering completely. I asked if we could start chemotherapy that afternoon.

The remainder of that day and the following were spent at the Marshfield Clinic, going from station to station, undergoing tests. I had a bone scan, CT scan, blood tests, ultrasound, MRI, x-rays, and mammograms. I was told by my doctor that weekly mammograms would not detect inflammatory breast cancer. I had always had my annual mammograms and nothing unusual was ever detected. MRIs are the best method for detecting this type of breast cancer. In fact, a mammogram of the left breast revealed no abnormality, even though my breast contained a tumor about six centimeters in diameter. And later, a mammogram of the right breast would reveal an abnormality when there was none. About 10 percent of mammograms are false positives or negatives, either of which can be distressing.

I was also told that no diagnostic equipment detected any spread, or “metastases” of the primary tumor. Yes! I was going to weather this storm. I would learn later that the equipment is imperfect and doesn’t detect everything, particularly tumors less than one centimeter in diameter.

My husband shared the news with our children. When I arrived home, my youngest daughter asked me, "Mom, are you going to die?" I replied, "I don't know that, Catherine. Only God knows that. But I want you to be assured that I will do all in my power to live because I'm not finished with you kids yet!"

On Wednesday, Oct. 6, I arrived at the clinic in the morning with my mother who had traveled to be with me. I was to receive a course of 16 weeks of chemotherapy treatment, or eight treatments every-other week. The first four were a mixture of Adriamycin and Cytoxan (lifetime doses) and the second four were Taxol. Although I don't like needles, I managed the IV in my hand. I came to look forward to my visits to the oncology department, because I knew I was in the hands of very competent staff, was always treated with the utmost dignity and respect, and was so well attended-to, being given a private room with a comfy overstuffed recliner and a television and bathroom. I always called my appointments, my "spa" treatments, because I said, "Where else can you go where they seat you comfortably, bring you a warm blanket, reading material, anything you want to eat or drink, wait on you hand and foot, and you don't have to answer the telephone?" It was my oasis from a hectic work environment.

I went home after about 3-4 hours, thinking, "I feel fine, that was a piece of cake. I can get through this." Just as surely as early evening arrived, so did the violent vomiting. I returned to the clinic that morning because I was dehydrated. I feel that was my biggest battle, attempting to remain hydrated. As simple as it sounds, taking in fluids or water, proved to be insurmountable. After each succeeding treatment, I would return to the clinic for several hours, to be rehydrated. Morphine was administered and we decided to use a different level of anti-nausea medication. Eating became a chore. I lost 30 pounds. My skin became very dry. Struggling to "feel good" was my primary aim. In addition to the ever-present nausea, I experienced restless leg syndrome, dry eyes, permanent neuropathy in my feet, loss of toe and fingernails, and the complete loss of my hair after the first treatment. My entire body felt as though it were shuddering. It hurt to move. Footsteps on carpeting sounded like pounding to me, and my husband removed the batteries from the chiming clock because I could not handle the noise. Additionally, I was extremely hot and didn't sleep much. A cousin came to visit me in the dead of winter and I greeted her at the door in my swimsuit! I also had to put my guests to bed, because I slept about two hours each night, and would fade in and out of sleep during the day when I was home. I spent long hours entertaining myself with humorous books and movies. I also listened to inspirational tapes and studied Bible passages on "healing," given to me by a church friend.

The physical changes in my body and to my appearance never bothered me. How significant is your hairstyle when you're facing death? After all, my body is just my "earthly shell." Cancer cannot rob me of my spirit and soul. I was shaken emotionally to the core a second time when I began to experience the outpouring of love, care and concern from everyone who were sent with perfect timing by God to minister to my every need.

I took to wearing very fashionable hats, all loaned to me by a girlfriend, and another girlfriend began to crochet "chemo caps" for me, and yet several other girlfriends knit caps for me. My hairdresser also fit me for a wig, which I wore less often, except to court. It doesn't matter what I do for a living, but I was, and still am, engaged full-time as a municipal lawyer. The court, my employer, and co-workers and my husband's co-workers were 100 percent there for me, accommodating my treatment schedule, and gifting me with a certificate to a restaurant delivery service. This act was also God-sent. The first thing you learn about facing this diagnosis and tackling treatment is that you are no longer in control. For someone who is used to "controlling" outcomes and directing others, the sense of complete loss of control over your life and your health is unbearable. When I couldn't stand to get to the kitchen to prepare a meal, my family was still fed.

I determined almost immediately that this new turn of events was something over which I had absolutely no control -- I could not "earn" or "buy" my recovery. And if it were to come at all, it would come at God's pace, not mine. For a first-born, over-achiever, this was especially frustrating. When people remarked that I seemed to be taking this news well, I replied, "What other choice do I have?" I don't know the outcome, but I am going to choose life and do everything within my power to live -- and the rest is up to God. I never felt angry with God, nor did I experience denial. Of course, there were anxious times --awaiting news of the results of tests, and "bad" days when I felt particularly sad. I never asked, "Why, me?" Life on earth is full of challenges, both good and bad, but it is how we accept these challenges and choose to react to them that determines our course and it is in giving all our burdens to God that we find peace.

The second-most frustrating aspect was the fact that I could not control how it affected those around me. My husband was never selfish enough to tell me how it affected him. Instead, he was there for me, playing countless games of Scrabble with me, attending all of my appointments with me and carefully discussing with the doctor our choices, as I couldn't remember what had been said, nor was I able to process the information in the same, rationale way he did. He would take me on long, silent rides as we just took in the sights and smells of the Wisconsin autumn -- the parks, rivers, trees and brilliant leaves changing colors – all without saying a word to each other. I also noticed around this time that I had a new set of "eyes" — a new appreciation for the simple, everyday things of life. I took in each sunset, noting the patterns of the clouds and the rays. I collected leaves. I noticed with a new clarity the innate beauty of the world in which we live. I had always hugged my children and told them that they were loved, but I began with regularity to tell others around me that I loved them. The personal slights we each experience in everyday life suddenly seemed petty and meaningless.

My dear husband also had to give me Neupogen injections (remember, I don't like needles) because my insurance would not pay for them to be injected by staff at the clinic. This meant that beginning two days after each chemotherapy treatment, I would receive an injection in alternating arms for eight consecutive days in an attempt to boost my white blood count. I received a total of 61 injections. Measures were taken to avoid close contact with the public. I received regular flu shots. I could not take chances with my already compromised immune system. I could not have a pap smear, a dental cleaning, or get in a motel pool or hot tub.

The course of chemotherapy treatment would be followed by surgery. This is directly opposite the treatment generally followed with other breast cancers. Surgery is generally performed, after which chemotherapy or radiation therapy is generally administered. In my case, due to the aggressive nature of the cancer, treatment is administered first to systemically bombard the body in an attempt to kill any cells that may have traveled to other parts of the body. No chances could be taken to perform surgery and wait for recovery to administer the chemotherapy drugs. This meant living with an extremely painful, swollen breast for four months while undergoing chemotherapy treatment.

I was told that five years ago almost no one survived this disease. When surgery was attempted first, the outcome was almost always death. I was told by one doctor that of all the cancers known to man, I had absolutely the worst kind and if it returned, there would be no recovery, but certain death.

Thus, I fell into an acceptable pattern of chemotherapy on Wednesdays, getting rehydrated on Thursday, and staying in bed on Friday, and most of the weekend, in an attempt to return to work on Monday. The weeks in between, I worked full time. I carefully calculated my sick leave bank, as I knew once all sick and vacation leave were exhausted, there would be no more income, perhaps no more job. I was in the fight for my life, and I wanted more than anything to be at work, to be useful, to be functioning efficiently. I wanted to focus on my work and family to maintain some sense of normalcy and to distract myself from darker thoughts.

Once I started receiving the Taxol, I would experience an intense burning in my hands and feet, as though they were being held over a fire, sometimes making it difficult to walk. This would set in around Friday afternoon, so I would literally spend the weekend in bed, just waiting out the symptoms, so I could return to work the following Monday. Some treatments were delayed if my white blood count was too low. My doctor would research very thoroughly my reported symptoms and would tell me that those were symptoms no one else reported. He also felt I was minimizing them, once saying, "You're willing yourself to heal, aren't you?"

Throughout this journey I felt intense loneliness, even though I was surrounded by well-meaning, caring, loving family, friends, co-workers and medical staff. I can't explain the reason for it. For one thing, I had never met anyone with inflammatory breast cancer, and to this day, have spoken with only two women by telephone, neither of which was also HER2-positive, like I was.

Around December, Dr. "S" informed me that a test had revealed that I was hormone receptor negative, putting me in another elite category of about 20 percent of all those with breast cancer. This meant in a nutshell, that the cancer was being fed not by hormones, but by an over expression of protein. On a scale of 0 to 3+, I was a "3+." This somehow added to the urgency of treatment and the need to be ever vigilant against this unwanted aggressor.

On Jan. 14, 2005, I celebrated the end of my chemotherapy treatment. With my husband at my side, and the entire staff congratulating me, I "rang the healing bell" and received a bottle of white grape juice. It was a beautiful moment.

God certainly works in mysterious ways. On Feb. 3, 2005, I had a modified radical left mastectomy. The staff person sent to prep me for surgery at the Marshfield Clinic turned out to be a high school classmate of mine. Discovering that connection gave me great personal comfort. My mother and husband were at my side again. I awoke from surgery around 4 p.m., and as this procedure is "outpatient" surgery, I was bundled into the car for an hour drive home around 10 p.m. My only sister, who resides in Texas, was on hand at home for a week to stand in for me. She has visited me every month of my illness since diagnosis, painting my kitchen, cleaning, cooking, and doing anything she could for me.

I returned to Marshfield, Wis. eight times over the next 16 days for follow-up care. A biopsy revealed two positive lymph nodes of the nine taken. Since the tumors were less than one centimeter in diameter, they were not detected by any diagnostic equipment just three weeks earlier. I felt as though this was bad news -- a setback -- and I felt the desperateness of my situation.

My husband informed me on one of our drives that he had been surfing the Internet. This was something I refused to do, because more often than not when I did that, I ended up feeling depressed. I would then remind myself that I am a unique person and only God knew what would happen to me. While my physicians operated on the best statistical evidence they possessed, they were just that -- statistics. I was going to be in the minority -- I was going to be a "survivor!" He told me uplifting stories posted on the Net about people who were "cured" (as opposed to being in "remission") and whose tests had revealed, "No evidence of disease." So they were

"NED." I remember that moment, thinking, I am going to tell everyone that I am "NED."

About this time I was also informed that I had both lobular and ductal carcinoma in situ — again, not particularly good news. I had quickly developed a burgeoning vocabulary shared by few others with whom I communicated, except my treating doctors and their staff.

I also came to learn that the blood tells us everything. A sense of dread began to creep in before each week's blood testing. There was something in my blood that made my doctor suspect that the cancer had spread to my bones, so another bone scan was ordered. I assumed at the time that the bone scan was "standard protocol" at that point in my treatment. The "result" at which my doctor was looking turned out to be attributable to the Taxol I was taking.

It seemed as though I was visiting the clinic 3-4 times per week. For several years, I probably hadn't visited a doctor more than once a year; now suddenly, the bulk of my time was spent in clinical settings, waiting rooms, exam rooms, chemo rooms. I was struck by two things: that there were always people in my midst who were far less fortunate than I was; and that I had begun to develop patience. I could sit for hours and not become agitated or angry or anxious waiting -- just waiting. I accepted my circumstances and asked God to give me the grace to handle them in ways familiar to me -- slowly, methodically, and with strength and faith.

On March 3, I began radiation therapy, daily except weekends, for a total of 25 treatments. This followed the preparation for radiation, which included "tattooing" with permanent ink the coordinates within which the radiation would be delivered. I agreed to be a guinea pig for "respiratory gaiting," a process by which the machine determines your breathing pattern, and delivers the radiation in between breaths, to minimize the effects to the heart and lung. Doctors practicing elsewhere in the state came to watch how this machine was used. It couldn't happen too soon. I was pushing for the radiation to start, as it had been one month and I needed to keep on going! The radiation was delivered deep into the left chest, as well as to the surface of the skin. I was told inflammatory breast cancer is like a skin cancer; it begins to grow along the chest wall initially and then spreads out from there. I suffered dry, burned skin toward the end of my treatment. I gave up Vicodin, my only painkiller, on Good Friday, as I didn't like the "mental fog" it produced.

By now, my veins had checked out. They were never very good, and on occasion several attempts had to be made to get an IV into my arm or top of my hand. In fact, when I awoke from surgery, the IV was in my left large toe. It was because of this increasing difficulty, that my doctor recommended a port be implanted, and so, on April 19, 2005, I had a port implanted near my right shoulder, through which blood would be drawn and fluids and chemotherapy administered.

Because I was HER2-positive, my doctor recommended Herceptin, a "miracle" drug that had been in clinical trial for some time, but which on the day I received it, appeared in the press, with facts about its astounding success in preventing recurrence. My doctor advised that he felt, "I had dodged a bullet," but thought the use of Herceptin, combined with another chemotherapy drug, was appropriate. The only drawback-- Herceptin decreases heart function-- so every nine weeks I had to have a MUGA scan. These were unpleasant only because as claustrophobic as I am, I needed varying levels of sedation to get through these exams, along with the MRI's and bone scans. I developed mental games of counting backwards from 1,000 by 3s or 5s or whatever I determined it would take to get me through a test of that length. My heart function was permanently decreased to a certain extent by the chemotherapy drugs earlier used, but throughout the use of Herceptin, my heart function remained stable and even increased slightly on one occasion.

My doctor used Navelbine with the Herceptin for the first six months of treatment. This drug was chosen because it did not cause hair loss and my hair was coming back -- although silver-white. I would have 53 weeks of weekly chemotherapy, beginning April 26, 2005 and ending April 24, 2006. I then went from every other week doctor visits and blood tests to once every three or four months, which was another mental adjustment, on top of "ending" treatment.

What if it came back? What would happen? Would it be caught soon enough?

At this time, I decided to pursue genetic counseling, which is not for the faint of heart. While I had no high risk factors for this disease, my mother's mother was diagnosed with colon cancer shortly before her death at 89, my mother's two maternal aunts and all her cousins, the four daughters of one aunt, all had breast cancer and half of them were gone. Neither my mother nor any of her four sisters had cancer. How could this be? I needed to know, one way or the other, whether I carried any of the detectable genetic markers which would tell me whether it was hereditary and if my own children had a 50 percent chance of having the same marker. I made several trips to Marshfield, Wis. and we collected the medical records of relatives, including my cousin, the oldest daughter of my dad's only brother, who lost her life in her early 50s to breast cancer. More good news came in June when we were told that my cancer was not hereditary, meaning that my children had no more likelihood of contracting cancer than the general population.

On Aug. 25, 2005, my world came crashing down when I discovered that my doctor had taken a new position and was leaving for St. Louis, MO. Selfishly, I felt lost, abandoned. I cried myself to sleep for two weeks. I could not fathom losing the one person to whom I had been tethered and upon whom I had come to depend to direct my recovery. He was so compassionate, so thorough, doing everything perfectly, I thought. Not too much information, nor too little. And then he invited me to let him know each year that I was still here. I do that on the anniversary of my diagnosis. And then I reminded myself that he had been there for me and seen me through the worst of my treatment, and others needed him.

Throughout that summer, Dr. "S" had taken special care to refer me to a dietician, a heart doctor and a gynecologist. My blood is still tested for the presence of markers for ovarian cancer. Further surgery was not warranted. I began studying what I could do in terms of exercise and diet to restore my health and boost my immune system. I was taking one prescription medication for an under active thyroid when I was diagnosed. Now, I was on iron and blood thinners because of my port. As those were removed from my regimen, I could include other foods. I read all that I could and attended presentations at the clinic by staff talking about diet. I began taking a regimen of vitamins and supplements around August of 2005, which I have faithfully maintained. I stopped drinking coffee and replaced it with green and white teas. I stopped drinking soda pop and began to drink water. I replaced most red meat with salmon and fish. I steam and broil -- in short, I wonder how I and my family survived with the eating habits and cooking I had heretofore thought healthy.

I was inspired after reading Lance Armstrong's books, and so I decided that rather than my birthday, it would be the anniversary of my survivorship that would be worth celebrating each year. Seriously -- does anyone you know look forward to turning 50? I could not wait to turn 50 on Sept. 22, 2005 -- no, I hoped I would live to see 50. That birthday came and went quietly, but on my anniversary on Oct. 4, I invited every woman who had been an instrumental part of my healing and recovery to my home. Of 49 invitations, 44 women came to my home in a thunderstorm to spend an evening chatting and rejoicing -- so that I could thank them for all they had done for me. That is still the one thought that can quickly reduce me to tears -- the generous, beyond-words show of unconditional love to me and my family, which was so humbling.

My treatment ended on May 8, 2006, when I underwent my second mastectomy. I understood intellectually that this surgery would not eradicate the possibility of the cancer returning, nor prevent a recurrence in my lungs, liver or bone, but I did it because it hurt as much as the first one and in so doing, I almost eliminated the possibility of the cancer returning to the breast tissue. There is always some remaining breast tissue, however small. I elected not to undergo reconstructive surgery, primarily because it is not important to me; it does not define who I am. I also would not undergo surgery for anything I did not perceive as life-threatening, and I was looking at multiple additional surgeries and more time lost from work. In fact, I had always considered breast reduction. I just never imagined my wish would be granted in this fashion! I was now free to be any size I wanted to be, or flat. No more bras and no more mammograms! It doesn't get much better than that.

Spiritually, I have always believed in God and felt his presence in my life. However, this experience has deepened my relationship with God. I prayed and talked to God constantly, and I still do. I felt His comforting presence with me at all times and felt assured I would be healed. I knew many people were praying for me and know that prayer works. Our prayers are heard. I attended a prayer group at my church and they laid hands on me and asked God to heal me. I cried little, because I never gave up hope; I had faith that God would heal me. I accepted my circumstances and asked for strength and grace to weather the storm. God refined me through this process, and brought me to a place where I was able to forgive freely, make peace with those from whom I had become separated, and look at the world through new eyes. I've reordered my priorities and let go of the little things.

Intellectually, I tried to educate myself and learn all I could about my cancer so that I could make the most informed decisions about my treatment. I chose the most aggressive treatment possible. I tried to make other women aware that they are the ones most attuned to their bodies and they should listen to them and seek medical attention without delay if their bodies told them something was wrong. Women with symptoms of the breast that mimic infection should know about inflammatory breast cancer and insist on an MRI or ultrasound. I met doctors who were unfamiliar with this type of cancer. I attended presentations of the cancer support group to learn all I could about cancer, and support my fellow patients. I came to record each of their names in my Bible so that I could remember to pray for each of them and their families by name.

Emotionally, I tried to stay strong for my family and focused on living and not on my situation. My faith in God and my belief that I would be healed gave me the presence of mind to continue. Once I relinquished control and gave my burden to God, I was able to function in a way that was limited only by my physical reaction to treatment.

Physically, I made a conscious effort to take better care of myself, resting often, drinking water, eating healthier, and getting massage therapy. My therapist was always a good friend, neighbor and master gardener. As soon as I fell ill, she would come to my house and put me to bed after a massage until I was well enough to leave the house. She planted my gardens for me and gave me pink flowers for my "pink" garden the following year.

What did I learn? Be thankful in all circumstances. I am not lucky, I am blessed. I am humbled to be employed, have health insurance and many supportive friends and family who sustained me and continue to do so. God is in control. Give all your cares to him. Be patient. Be forgiving. Tell those you love that you love and appreciate them and show it. Choose life! Appreciate all things. Choose to live your life with a cheerful heart; it is much more pleasant and productive than living with doubt, worry, melancholy, or anger.

There is life after cancer and cancer treatment! Our bodies are changed in irrevocable ways, but our souls are intact and our spirits strong.

“Mom”
By Leslie Jacobson (Anne’s daughter)

Stay strong,
It will not be that long.

Have no fears,
God is always near.

May I be sensitive like a dove
And give you all of my love.

I know you may get blue,
But just remember that
All of your friends are true.

Everyone will stand by your side,
And help you through this difficult ride.

To us, you mean so much
All the way down to your touch.

So take care and believe,
And oh, I promise you will be relieved.

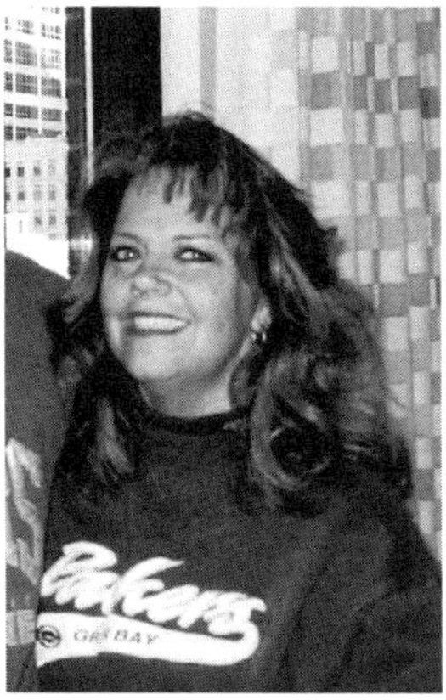

Chapter Fifteen

Out of the Box

By Sondra Clinkscales, Winona, MN

My name is Sondra Clinkscales, I am a Green Bay Packers fan and I am a breast cancer survivor (probably in that order). Though I have been in remission for six years, breast cancer is with me every day. Someone once asked me if going through the experience of overcoming breast cancer makes you feel different. I tell them if taking your breast out of a box every morning and putting it on before you go to work makes you "different," then, well I suppose that I am.

It has often been said that life is a series of experiences that together, help to define you and shape your existence. Growing up in a small Minnesota town with four brothers and sisters, my life has always been defined by family. As a devoted daughter of a die-hard Green Bay Packers fan, my days were often spent watching football with my dad, joining his cheering section as each and every year we hoped for the big win. Living in Minnesota, my father went against the odds and stayed true to the Wisconsin Green and Gold, sticking with the rivals across the river throughout their ups and downs as a team. I suppose you could say that I inherited his loyalty and his love for the game, for I too am a die-hard Green Bay fan. Some people might say that I bleed green and gold. I just tell them it's genetic; I must have inherited it from my dad.

Just as the Green Bay Packers shaped my youth and gave me something to fight for, in a strange way, cancer has shaped my existence, striking a blow to my family in so many ways, and shifting my priorities, all the while teaching me what it means to fight.

As a young child, I learned that cancer was the awful illness that made my Aunt Dorothy sick. She was diagnosed with breast cancer in her early thirties while she was pregnant with her third child, a beautiful baby girl. The doctors performed a radical mastectomy immediately after her delivery, fearing that without the surgery, she wouldn't live to see her children grow up.

I remember making the big trip to Chicago with my family to visit her shortly after the baby was born. A few days into our stay, I accidentally walked in on her while she was breastfeeding my new baby cousin. I couldn't help but stare as she nursed her newborn daughter with her one healthy breast, while a four inch scar took the place of where her other breast should have been. As a child, I probably didn't realize the significance of this moment, but I look back on it now and see the dichotomy of life and death, sickness and health, and the human body's ability to provide in the face of sickness. I know now that the emotional scars left by her illness were far deeper than the physical ones.

My aunt succumbed to breast cancer two short years later, leaving behind three young children and a husband. As a child myself, so dependent on my mother's care both physically and emotionally, it seemed incomprehensible how a mother could be taken away from her children when they needed her so much. It seemed so abrupt, almost without warning. Later I would come to understand that cancer often happens that way, and that if you look hard enough, you can see the beauty in the face of the adversity it brings.

As an adult, cancer took its toll on my immediate family some years later when my 40-year-old brother, Matthew, was diagnosed with stage four colon cancer and was forced to undergo chemotherapy. My brother, a grown man with two of his own small children at home, had to fight a battle similar to the one that my aunt had lost.

Matthew's cancer was a shock to my family. "But he's so young," we would say. "He takes care of himself. How can this happen?" In a way, cancer is the great equalizer. It can happen to the old and young, those that appear healthy and those plagued with a lifetime of illness.

Matthew's cancer was incredibly difficult for my mom and dad to deal with. As parents, we want to shield our children from life's perils, no matter what their age. I think my parents questioned their own health and felt that their son was somehow cheated, that the illness should have been their burden.

Life is a series of ebbs and flows, and through the years of watching the Packers win and lose but never go to the Super Bowl, my dad would often say, "I sure would like to see the Packers win a Super Bowl before I die." His wish came true in January 1997, when his beloved team won the championship. Sadly, his time to relish in the victory was cut short.

The day after their Super Bowl win, while Matthew was still undergoing chemotherapy, my mom called me and said to come quick, she thought Dad was having a stroke. I raced to their house to get my father to the hospital. In a matter of hours we received some devastating news. My dad had cancer and it had spread throughout his entire body. The tumors in the brain were affecting his speech, creating stroke-like symptoms. He was told to go home, put his house in order, and say goodbye to his family. Life can change in an instant, and in this case it did.

My two sisters and I set up camp at my parent's home, and spent our days and nights helping our mom take care of Dad, allowing him to live the rest of his life in the comfort of his home, surrounded by the family that loved him. Dad died six weeks later, fighting with everything he had until he was finally ready to say goodbye. I believe that his fighting spirit inspired my brother to beat the odds in the battle against his own illness. Ten years have since passed and Matthew is still in remission.

One year after my father's passing my mom was diagnosed with colon cancer. My father must have been watching over us during this time, because Mom was able to do what he couldn't. She fought bravely and won, and is still in remission today.

Three of the people that mean most to me battled cancer, and through it I lost my father. I spent a great deal of time trying to figure out why this had happened, and then realized that I had to find a better outlet for my frustration and anger. I decided to give my time to organizations dedicated to cancer research and treatment and aid in their fundraising efforts. Organizations like the LeRoy Butler Foundation.

Early on in my fundraising, it became apparent that those who would give generously did so because they could put a name and a face on their contribution. Often they had a friend or family member who was dealing with the illness. Then there were those who would decline to donate, claiming they didn't know anyone with cancer. To them I would smile politely, muttering under my breath, "Did you ever open your eyes? They're everywhere!" People don't have to look ill or be bald to have cancer. Some of the most vibrant people that I knew -- even those in my own family -- had it. They just chose not to dwell on it or be defined by their illness. I believe that the desire to educate people about how pervasive cancer can be kept me motivated to raise money for such a worthy cause.

Then in 2000, everything changed in an instant. I found out I had breast cancer. I like to joke that everyone in my family had colon cancer so I had to be original, to go out and find my own type. I guess you could say it found me. During a routine breast exam, I discovered a reddish-colored lump the size of a walnut on my right breast. Given my family history, I was concerned and made an appointment with my doctor. After a mammogram, ultrasound and biopsy, the doctor told me the lump was fibercystic and nothing to worry about, but the concern was another area of my breast. I had what was called carcinoma in situ, a very serious form of breast cancer.

I'll never forget what the doctor said as she delivered the diagnosis. "If you were my daughter I would advise you to have the breast removed," she said. I remember looking up and seeing a picture of her beautiful daughters and realizing what she really meant. It was as if she said, "Don't fool with this, and don't jeopardize your life."

In keeping with the fighting spirit of my family, I decided to have a back-to-back procedure done. My doctor would remove my breast and a plastic surgeon would put in an expander so that I would be able to have an implant inserted at a later date.

The day of my surgery I was so nervous, completely clueless as to what was in store. The doctor assured me that this was a routine procedure, that I would feel nothing. I remember how cold and scared I felt -- not sure if I would be able to identify with the version of myself that would come out of the operating room. As women, we're so defined by the physical; we're a sum of our parts, and the possibility of losing one creates a deep and overwhelming feeling of loss.

After surgery my first memory was screaming in the recovery room, feeling extreme pain despite the doctor's assumptions to the contrary. I just wanted to get out. I wanted to go home and see my husband and my children, to be free from the confines of a hospital bed. At about 3 a.m. I began asking the nurses in the hospital if they'd let me go home today. "I WANT TO GO HOME!" I would yell, making my demands to whomever would listen.

The doctor came in to check on me -- I told her I was ready to go home, drainage tubes and all. Call it my incredible social skills or infinite powers of persuasion (or the fact that the entire medical staff just wanted to get the annoying, whining lady as far away as possible), but I was discharged that afternoon.

My post-surgery homecoming brought an unbelievably good feeling. It felt fantastic to be home in my own little comfort zone. My husband, Rick, made every effort to make our home recovery-friendly, decorating the bedroom with flowers and creating a sense of warmth, a safe haven that would somehow protect me from the tumultuous procedure I had undergone. My husband truly amazed me through the entire ordeal. From his thoughtful welcome home to the compassion and empathy that he showed when looking at me for the first time after surgery, his patience and grace brought new meaning to the term "unconditional love."

Like most women faced with a life-changing alteration to their body, I was undoubtedly concerned with what I would find when the bandages were removed. I had heard so many horror stories from breast cancer survivors about how their husbands were put off by the scars -- not wanting anything to do with them. In my case it was the opposite. My husband was my supporter, my caregiver, listener and my shoulder to cry on. I cried many times around him and I'm sure he got sick of seeing me cry, but he never showed it. I may have lost my breast, but my heart was full of love for a husband who looked past the suffering and saw me -- really saw me.

When it came time to take off the bandages and unveil my missing breast, the fear of what was beneath the white gauze overcame me. My husband and I made a deal. He agreed to examine it first and let me know how my newly changed body looked. If he gave the go-ahead, I would muster up the courage to take a look for myself.

When he peeled back the layers of gauze and tape and took a long look, he had absolutely no reaction. His calm demeanor persuaded me to look too, and I found that my scar was nothing compared to the image that I had created in my mind. We still laugh today at my reaction. The first thing I said was, "Well, it looks like a collapsed muffin!" Somehow, my ability to compare the results of this major life-changing surgery to a botched baking attempt lightened the mood in the room. At that moment, I knew that I would be OK.

Restlessness started to settle in a few days after I came home from the hospital. I wanted desperately to return to my normally active lifestyle, despite the obvious need for my body to heal. I wanted to go out with friends and socialize and be normal like everyone else, but I had two drainage tubes coming out of my chest. My husband, the handiest man I know, went to the hardware store and bought me a carpenter's nail pouch. We put each of the two drainage bags into a compartment of the nail pouch, covered me in an oversized sweatshirt to conceal it and headed out for a night with friends. Nobody suspected the makeshift apparatus hidden beneath my clothes, and most importantly, I had fun that night!

Soon after the surgery, I began to make regular visits to a plastic surgeon for saline fills that would expand the skin and make room for the implant that would eventually be inserted. Each time I went for a saline fill, my chest grew tighter and left me feeling uncomfortable and in severe pain. I told my doctor that something was wrong, but he was always in too much of a hurry to concern himself with my discomfort. I remember one instance when he was leaving on a trip to Alaska and pushed the saline fill process at a rapid rate in order to wrap up the appointment and make his plane. I wondered what was more important, his Alaskan fishing trip or my physical comfort. Apparently there was no contest between me and the fish he hoped to catch. Let's just say the fish won. Little did I know that his carelessness would end up causing me more pain than the entire surgical process I had already undergone.

Well guess what happened? You've got it - I split it open like the back end of a pair of pants. My local doctor couldn't fix the rip in my chest, so against my better judgment I returned to the plastic surgeon responsible for the saline fills. My surgeon took out the ill-fitting expander, but stitched the incision improperly, leaving me with a very dangerous case of staph infection. That was my last encounter with the surgeon with the penchant for Alaskan wildlife. I headed back to the doctor who conducted my mastectomy operation for a consultation.

The staph infection was pervasive, seemingly determined to stick with me, despite my best attempts to kill it. I remember my young son stuffing a foot of tape into the hole in my chest to help rid my body of the staph. Nothing seemed to work. My doctor worked tirelessly to clear up the infection, but quickly acknowledged that the seriousness of it was beyond her expertise. She recommended a plastic surgeon, who she thought to be the best in the state, and I believe he was. He cleaned up the staph infection immediately, continuing treatment until I was completely healed. Had I known then what I know now, I would never have jumped at the first surgeon recommended to me. I would have searched for a surgeon with an impeccable reputation. My health, as I have learned through a struggle to regain it, is priceless.

Six years later the cancer is gone and I'm living a happy and healthy life, surrounded by family and friends, the people who mean the most to me. Now that time has passed and I have gained some emotional distance from the roller coaster experience of surgery and the struggle to heal, I'm considering having reconstruction done to fix my chest and to allow room for an implant. I just want to feel normal and have two breasts like most other women. Luckily, I work for a clothing manufacturer, so whenever I need an extra one in the meantime, there are always plenty of shoulder pads lying around.

My personal experience with breast cancer, as well as the way that cancer has pervaded my family, has shaped me in ways that I could never have imagined. I have always had a strong faith in God, but the experience of illness showed me the unsuspecting ways in which God can work miracles. I asked God to help me through my time of need and I believe He did. I learned very quickly to have faith and stop dwelling on things that were beyond my control. The lesson it taught was as much about fighting the illness as coming to terms with it -- accepting life's struggles and embracing the journey. This lesson was a lifetime in the making, but it took the prospect of losing life to really grasp it.

Life is cyclical, and the fond memories I have for my father and the time we spent watching the Green Bay Packers inspired me to begin working to raise money for the LeRoy Butler Foundation. LeRoy, a former Packer, is such an inspiration. The way that he could fire up a crowd was and still is so inspiring to us, the fans, and his team. His commitment to the breast cancer cause and his ability to use his high profile position to generate awareness inspired me to lend a hand. The LeRoy Butler Foundation is an inspiration, and I feel very lucky to be able to do my part to help LeRoy raise funds and awareness for a cause that is so close to my heart.

My name is Sondra Clinkscales, I am a Green Bay Packers fan and I am a breast cancer survivor.

A woman's breast
By Christine Kennelly, Sondra's sister

Attributes are endless and adjectives abound, and because of this women are devastated when they have to excise this part of themselves. I really understand the sense of loss. We are overwhelmed in literature, art and the media with that part of the female anatomy. History of art and literature shows the reverence, but the media of today has us doing surgical acrobatics to be bigger and better.

We as a society have bought into this vain concept that we can be more with a nip and a tuck. All these women want is the semblance of what they once had, a continuum of self.

Wouldn't it be wonderful if we felt as strongly about the intangible as the tangible? As a representative of the race of women, I would rather be glorified for courage, grace and perseverance than a D cup size. The women that go through these surgeries have these characteristics and more. Why don't we start seeing them -- really seeing them?

Afterword

It has been a privilege to have worked with the women whose stories are presented in this book. During the time it took to compile the chapters, I was able to get to know many of the women, and I certainly spent a lot of time with each their stories.

While all of the stories are very different and unique, there are certain themes that I found running throughout this whole book. The first is that we all need to be strong advocates for our own health and our bodies. We cannot leave the responsibility for our health up to someone else. Another lesson is that our healthcare system needs help. These stories must be told in order to make changes in the way prevention, testing and care is carried out. The fears and concerns of all patients need to be taken seriously and addressed.

In a twist of irony, right in the midst of working on the chapters, I discovered a lump in my right breast. I was haunted by the stories I was working on, yet felt hopeful because these women were so inspiring. For about two weeks I went through many of the same emotions these women describe. The wondering, the questions, the fear and the imagined scenarios. This lump turned out to be a simple cyst, but it certainly made me much more empathic, and it was a not so gentle reminder to live life to its fullest. We just never know.

Inspiration comes in many forms; I hope some will find inspiration through the pages of this book. For myself, that insight came through a simple story of stones and water. A young child was throwing stones into a lake. His grandfather came along and jokingly said if he kept at it the water level would rise. Curious, this young boy kept throwing more and more stones with a watchful eye on the lake. His grandfather chuckled and explained that although he would see ripples from the stones, he would never actually be able to see the change in the water.

That story hit home. We all can make ripples, which can make waves, which over time change the water level – but if we just stand there watching the lake, we'll never see the water level rise. The same is true in the quest to beat cancer and the support of those with cancer. Big changes start with little ripples and every ripple contributes to the bigger picture. So I challenge everyone to go out there, and in your own way, start making ripples, even though you may never see the water level rise.

My thanks go out to Mary Beth Bockhorst for her talents in designing the book cover, Jean Militello and Jo Ann Wahlen for proofing, Kym Lindau for her hard work, Marshall Cook for his wisdom and Jill Huizenga and Denise Fitzsimmons for their support. And many thanks go out to all the women who over the years have been models of inspiration for all of us.

Peace,
Renee Wahlen Tillema
August 2007

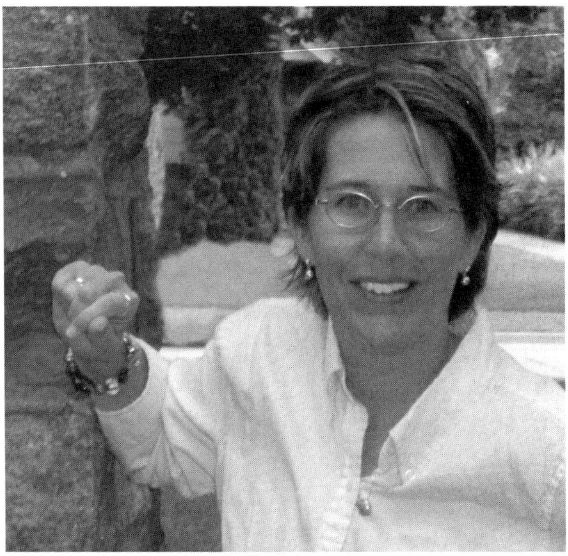

Renee Wahlen Tillema is the editor for InSpire Magazine (*www.inspiremag.biz*), a regional women's publication based in Wisconsin. She is also owner of Nuance Creative Writing, LLC (*www.nuancewriting.com*), a writing service for businesses, organizations and non-profits. Renee lives in Beaver Dam, Wis. with her family.

Final thoughts

I have had the great pleasure to work with LeRoy Butler organizing speaking engagements and various appearances for him in the Fox Valley area, ranging from elementary schools to large local companies. I have gotten to know LeRoy on both a professional and personal level. I can say without a doubt that he is the kindest, most generous person I know. He truly cares about people.

He is a rare individual who would use the fact that he is famous to help women who are stricken with a terrible disease. It is one thing to help someone you love, a family member or a close friend, emotionally and financially. But to use his celebrity status to help people he does not know, is a very special person indeed.

I am honored and proud to have been a small part of this book, and to be able to call LeRoy my friend.

Bev Van Geffen

The LeRoy Butler Foundation for Breast Cancer has raised over $300,000 that is used for research, financial assistance, treatment costs, and public education on breast cancer.

Your interest in helping fight breast cancer makes us teammates in the struggle. Together, we can make a difference.

Additional copies of this book can be purchased through the LeRoy Butler Foundation. For more information visit: www.leroybutlerfoundation.org

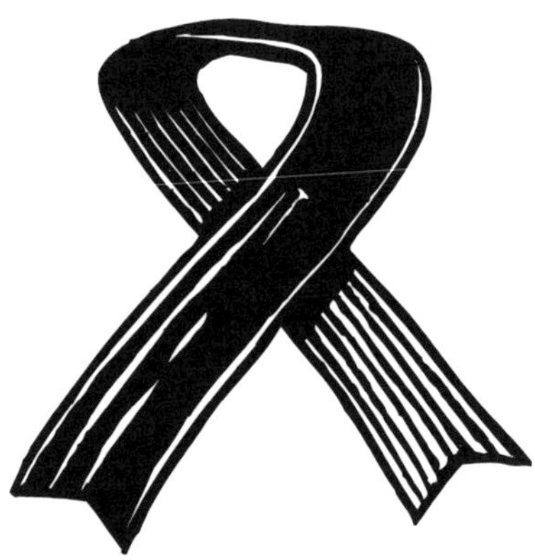